Solutions for Dental Esthetics
The Natural Look

Toyohiko Hidaka

Solutions for Dental Esthetics

The Natural Look

Toyohiko Hidaka

What we see with our eyes is not all there is to see.
Repeated experience is necessary to reveal the whole.

Quintessence Publishing Co. Ltd.
London, Berlin, Chicago, Tokyo, Barcelona, Istanbul, Milan, Moscow, New Delhi, Paris, Peking, Prague, São Paulo and Warsaw

Title of the original edition:
Solutions for Dental Esthetic
Look the Nature

The dental laboratory work pictured in this book was prepared by:
Satoshi Tsuchiya
Koichi Hirao
Takahiro Wakui
Koji Aida
Ken Takahashi
Toshia Shimogori
Toshiyuki Ebisuzaki

This book was developed in collaboration with:
Norio Itahashi: a/h Studio
Second Department of Dental Prosthetics, Tsurumi University School of Dental Medicine
(Chief: Prof. Toshio Fukushima)

British Library Cataloguing in Publication Data

Hidaka, Toyohiko
Solutions for dental esthetics : the natural look
1. Dentistry - Aesthetic aspects
I. Title
617.6

ISBN-13: 9781850971764

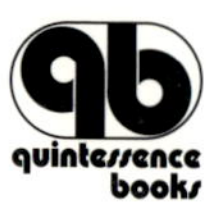

Quintessence Publishing Co, Ltd
Grafton Road, New Malden, Surrey KT3 3AB,
Great Britain
www.quintpub.co.uk

Printed in Germany

Foreword

A beautiful person, an attractive face – these certainly are and have been things of great appeal and interest since the historical beginnings of civilization in the Eastern world as well as in the Western world. But what is beauty? The concept of beauty can vary from one part of the world and from one period of history to another. Although the Japanese perception of beauty had been completely different from that of other societies for ages, it has changed significantly over the course of time. As Hiroto Murasawa indicated in his book "The Cultural History of the Face", the teeth used to be a minor factor in the perception of beauty in Japan compared to the contour of the face or the shape of the eyes and the nose. Before the opening of Japan to the rest of the world (Meiji Renovation), blackening of the teeth was a custom practised by married women of the educated class. The purpose was to make the teeth as inconspicuous as possible. In contrast, clear pupils and white teeth were very important factors in the Chinese concept of beauty.

After the Second World War and, in particular, in the last ten years, the Japanese ideals of beauty transformed radically, and the mouth has become a focus of esthetic attention. The Japanese were often disparaged because of their "unattractive" mouths. This created an invisible barrier when the internationalization of Japan began. The Japanese had a reserved nature that was written on their faces whereas they encountered a Western culture that was much more expressive. Japan assimilated without regard to the potential consequences. Former U.S. Secretary of State Henry Kissinger is rumored to have said that Japanese politicians' mouths stink. This unpleasant and embarrassing statement is a case in point.

Cosmetic modification of appearance is relatively easy to achieve by dying the hair, applying creative makeup, or piercing the nose or the ears. The result is that everyone looks alike. However, it is not so simple to change the physical shape of the jaw or teeth. A dentist with a fine sense of esthetics combined with a high level of professional competence must be found for this task. At this point, it is legitimate to ask whether the current state of dentistry in Japan is adequate for proper esthetic restoration of the mouth and teeth of the Japanese people. In dental practice in this country, it was not long ago that shiny metal on the front teeth, gingivitis and nicotine stains were not considered to be problematic. Therefore, a rapid change is not to be expected.

Furthermore, with a treatment approach that aims for average results, many problems remain. Reconstructive treatment of dental and facial malformations has reached a respectable level due to close collaboration between orthopedic and surgical specialists. It is now an established and reliable concept. However, since this treatment approach only achieves average results, it does not necessarily produce an esthetically acceptable result for each individual patient. Therefore, we must ask again: "What exactly constitutes beauty?" Precisely this legitimate question could be a useful starting point for esthetic dentistry.

Dr. Hidaka is a conscientious dentist who defines the beauty of the Japanese based on professional experience and on state-of-the-art technologies such as those used in implantology, prosthetics and periodontology, but also and especially based on harmony between the shape of the face and the personality and perceptions of the individual patient. With this photographic atlas, he attempts to cultivate a sense of esthetics through pictures that speak their own language without many words. There is no simple rule of thumb for producing beauty. Dr. Hidaka has intentionally avoided this impression. Instead, his book demonstrates a more differentiated and sensitive approach derived from the collective sum of his esthetic knowledge. To the reader, I recommend that you allow yourself to be inspired to create the esthetic dentistry of the future.

Kanichi Seto
Member of the Science Council of Japan
Dean, Tsurumi University School of Dental Medicine

Foreword

A book of hitherto unknown free and groundbreaking design has been published! Its descriptive format provides a flexible response to that which the individual reader would like to see and explore. The informative content of the book, which conveys rules for the integration of esthetic elements in daily practice, is outstanding for two reasons: Firstly, because it is based on scientific studies and investigations, it provides a basis for the scientific evaluation of dental esthetics. Secondly, it analyzes the characteristics of natural teeth according to age. Toyohiko Hidaka has compiled a tremendous amount of photographic material for this purpose. Hence, the book is extremely useful for producing age-specific esthetic restorations for the individual patient.

To my knowledge, this is the first such book that collates scientifically based esthetic data and documents difficult-to-obtain information about the characteristics of natural teeth across all age ranges.

The effort that Dr. Hidaka has invested in this book in addition to the many tasks in his busy professional schedule has certainly come to full fruition.

Masao Yamazaki
President of the International Society of Japan Clinical Dentistry (SJCD)
Chairman of SJCD Tokyo

Preface

The goal of any dental treatment is to maintain the function and health of the teeth and gums. The functional and healthy stomatognathic system of the human body is natural and beautiful. Esthetic dentistry is not a special area of dental medicine, but rather is a conception of dentistry that attempts to find uncompromising solutions to problems down to the last details. Concepts of beauty change with time; moreover, they are culture-dependent and subject to subjective perceptions. Hence, the esthetic dentist must always attempt to create the realization of beauty according to the wishes of the individual patient. This book was written with the intent of providing patients and dentists, with different conceptions and wishes, various points of reference along the way towards a common goal.

Perfect symmetry does not exist in nature. The beauty created by nature is perfect imperfection. Symmetry and balance are, however, very important factors in facial esthetics because many patients who wish to have an ideal facial appearance consider these characteristics to be essential. As esthetic dentists, we have an obligation to create oral and dental restorations that meet the expectations of the patient and which are perceived by the patient as pleasant.

Toyohiko Hidaka

Contents

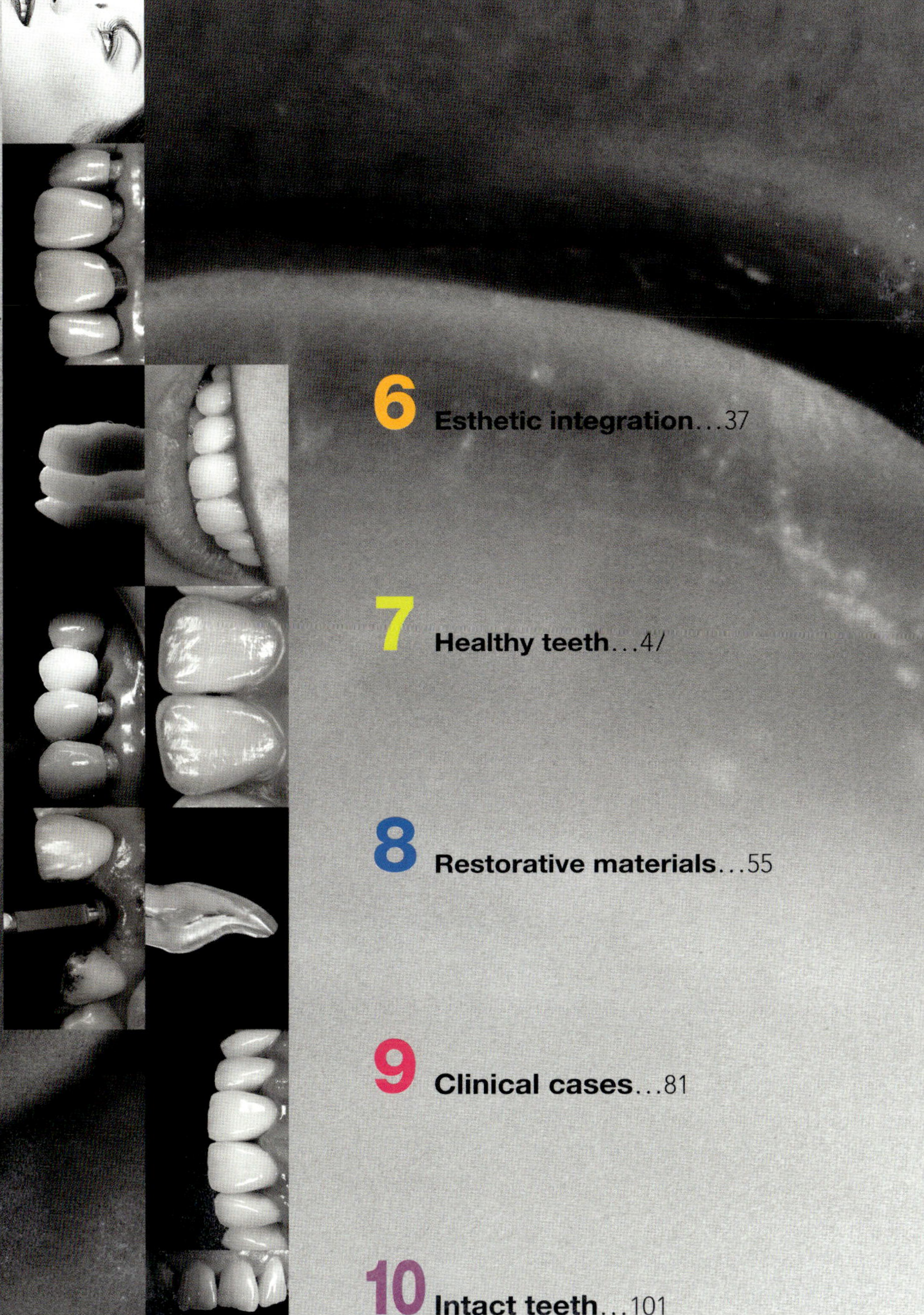

Illustrations marked with a red square ■ originally appeared in the sources cited on page 145.

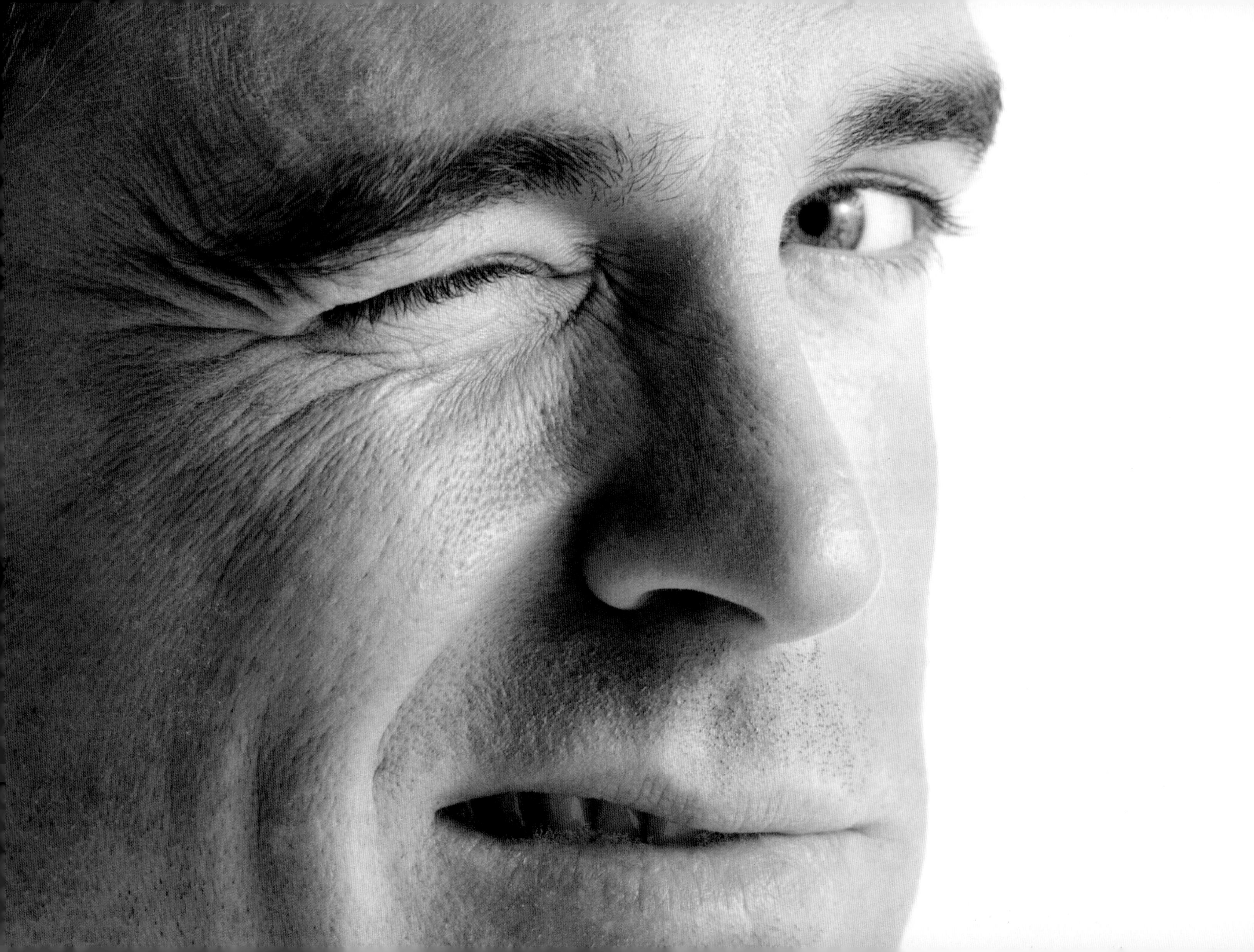

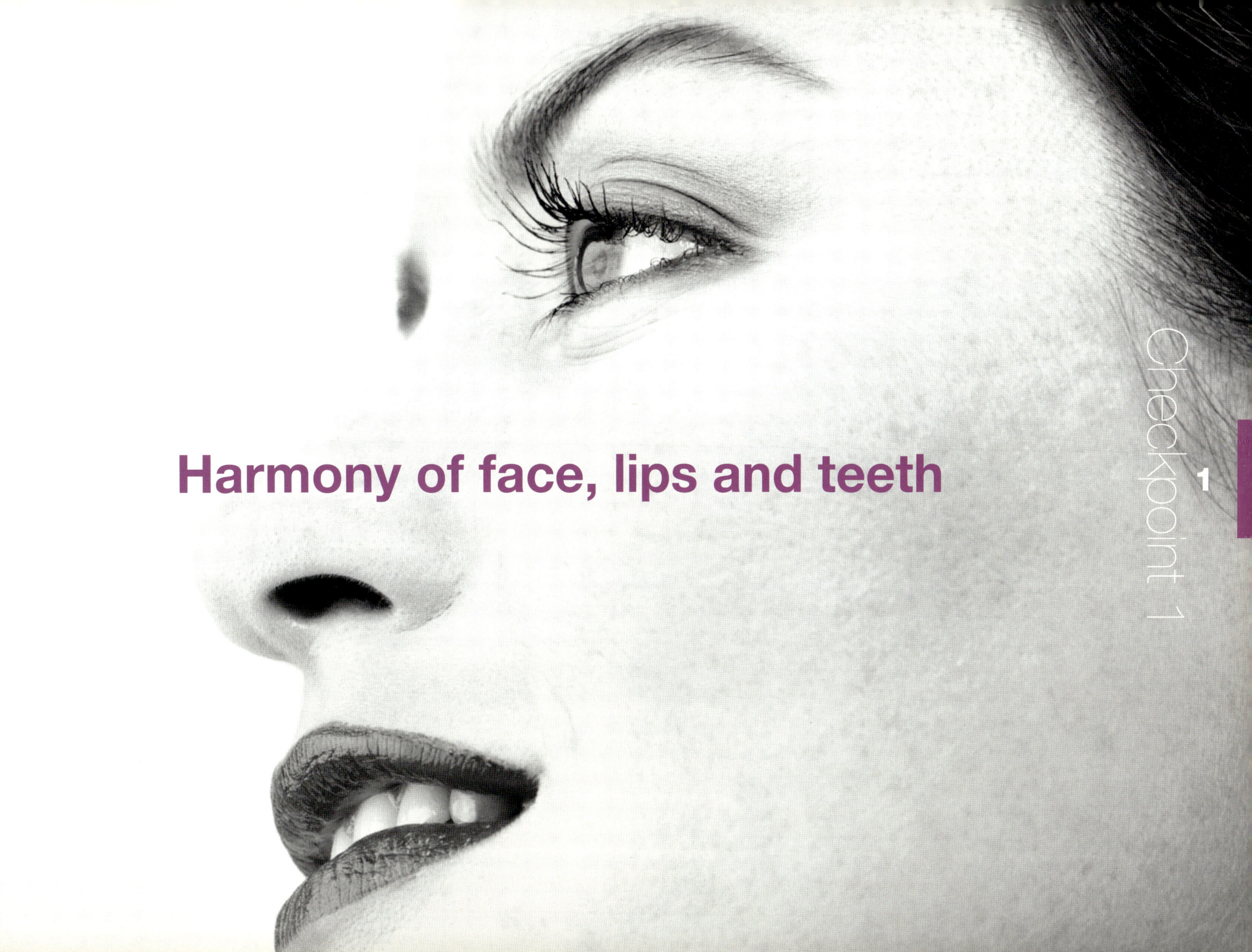

Harmony of face, lips and teeth

Checkpoint 1

Before starting a restorative treatment, the first step of the esthetic analysis is to evaluate the relationships between the face, lips and teeth.

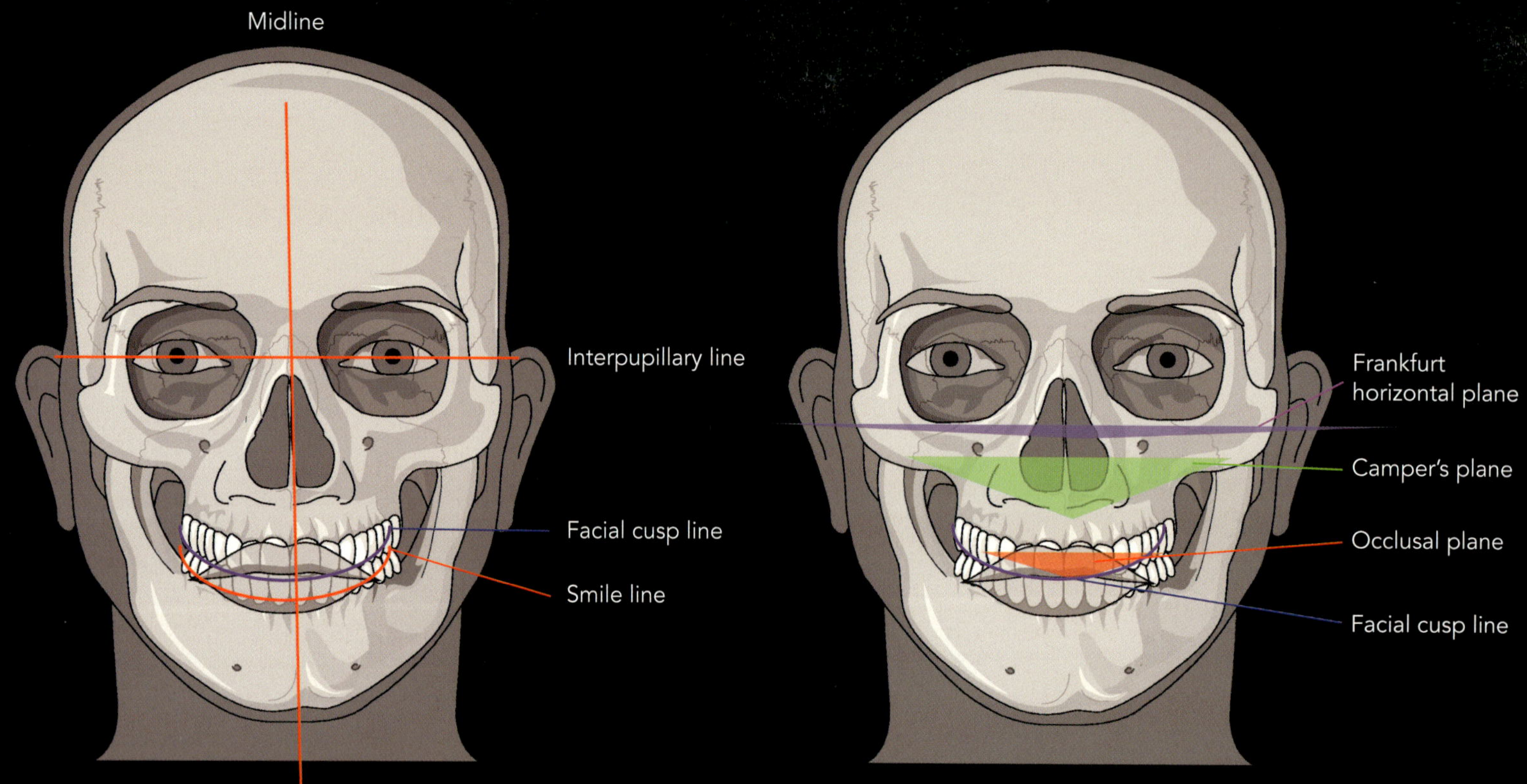

Frontal view (facial evaluation)

It is esthetically desirable to have an interpupillary line that runs perpendicular to the facial midline and parallel to the smile line. The facial cusp line is the imaginary line that extends parallel to the smile line and connects the incisal edges of the anterior teeth with the cusp tips of the posterior teeth. Creating this line is the goal of esthetic restoration.

Frontal view (facial evaluation)

Since the facial cusp line lies in the occlusal plane, it extends virtually parallel to Camper's plane or turns slightly downward dorsally. Relative to the Frankfurt horizontal plane, it rises dorsally about 8 to 12 degrees.

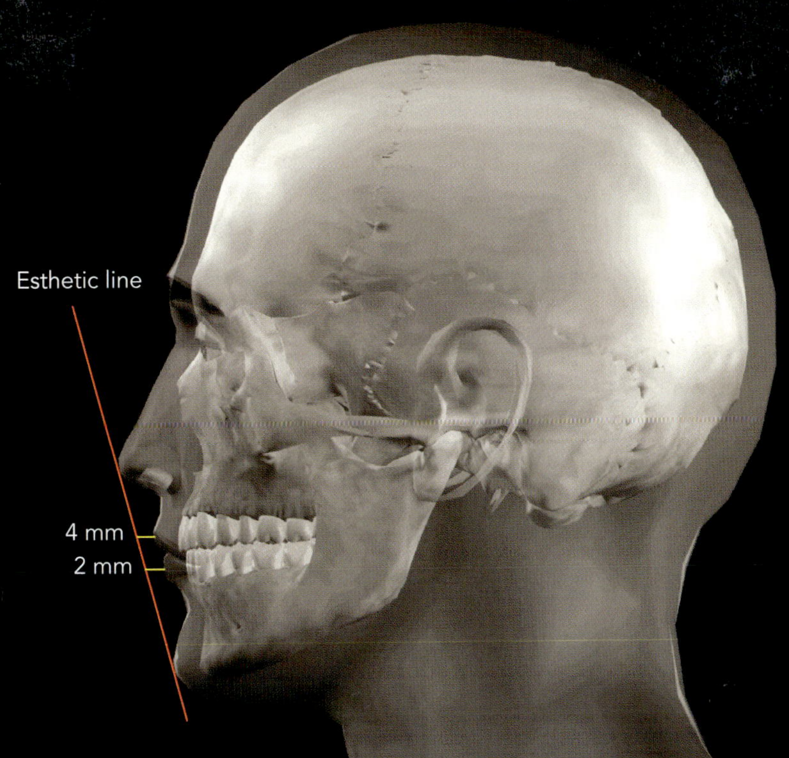

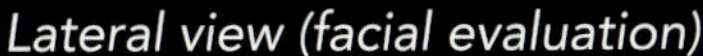

Lateral view (facial evaluation)

According to Ricketts, esthetic balance is achieved when the distance between the line connecting the tip of the nose and chin (esthetic line) and the line connecting the upper and lower lip is approximately 4mm and 2 mm, respectively.

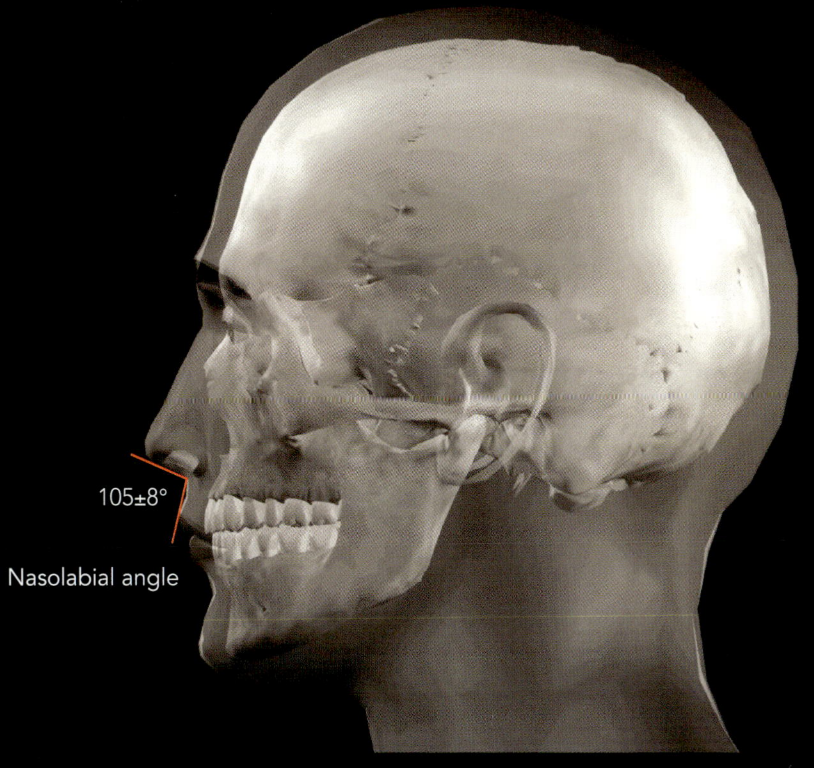

Lateral view (facial evaluation)

According to Olwyn, the average nasolabial angle is 102 degrees. However, 105 ± 8 degrees should be used as the angle of reference for Japanese subjects.

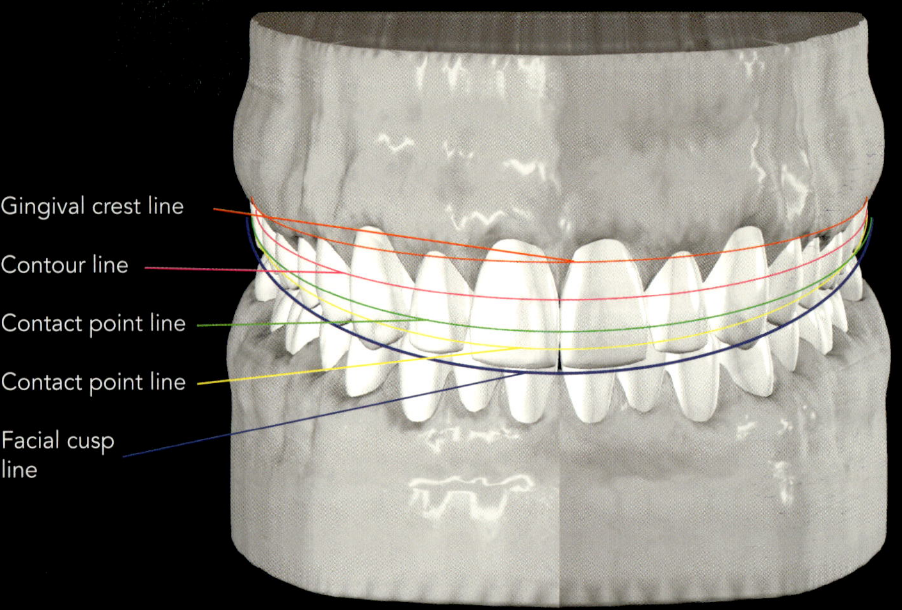

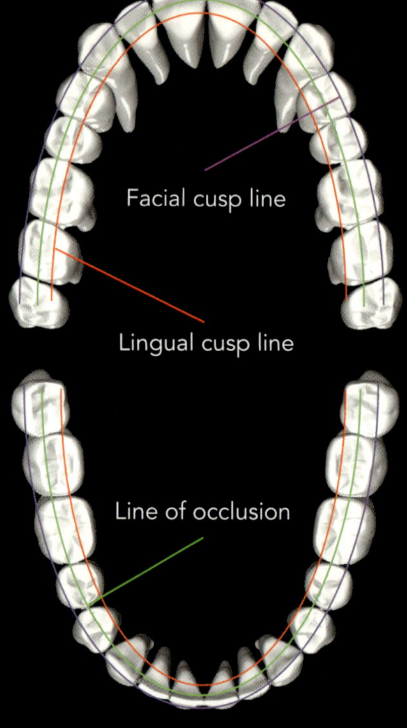

Frontal imaginary lines

Ideally, the gingival crest line (the line connecting the highest points of the gingival margin), the contour line (the line connecting the highest points of the buccal bulges of the dental crowns), the contact point line (the line connecting the contact points), the marginal ridge line (the line connecting the incisors and the peaks of the marginal ridges of the posterior teeth of the maxilla) and the facial cusp line should be parallel to one another.

Occlusal imaginary lines

In the occlusal view, the line of occlusion (line connecting the central fossa, the occlusal contact points in the fissures of the posterior teeth, the occlusal contact points of the anterior teeth) and the lingual cusp line (line connecting the lingual cusps of the posterior teeth and the lingual tuberculae of the anterior teeth) should extend analogous to the facial cusp line (the line connecting the buccal cusps of the posterior teeth and the incisal edges of the anterior teeth).

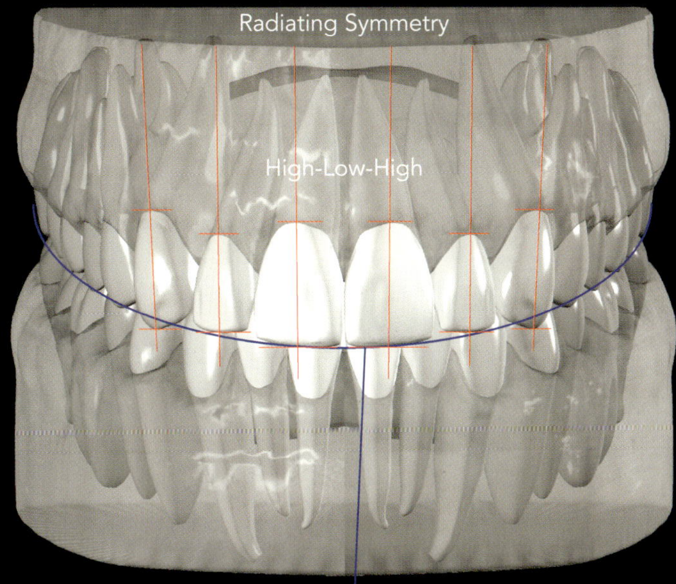

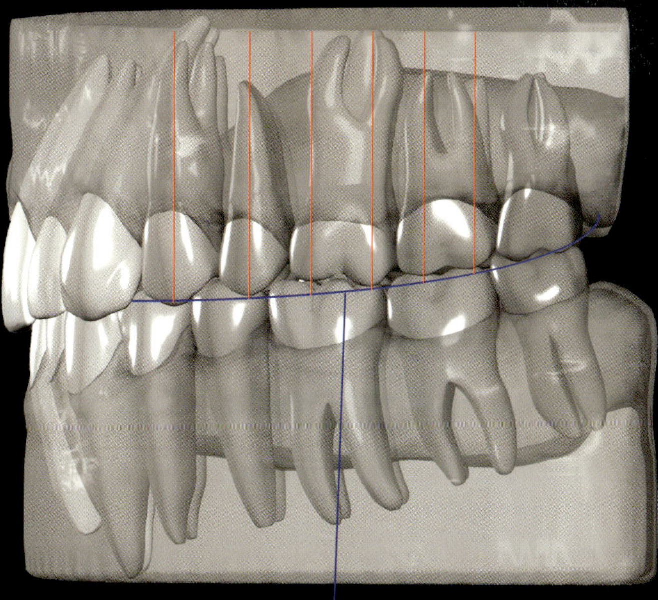

Axis of the anterior teeth
Incisal and gingival height

Unlike the true axis, the imaginary axis of the anterior teeth deviates cranially from midline (radiating symmetry). The incisal and cervical sections of the lateral incisors are shorter than the central incisor and canine teeth. It is therefore esthetically ideal to have the anterior teeth form a high-low-high pattern.

Axis of the posterior teeth

The axes of the crowns of the posterior teeth are almost identical with the true tooth axes, and they run perpendicular to the facial cusp line.

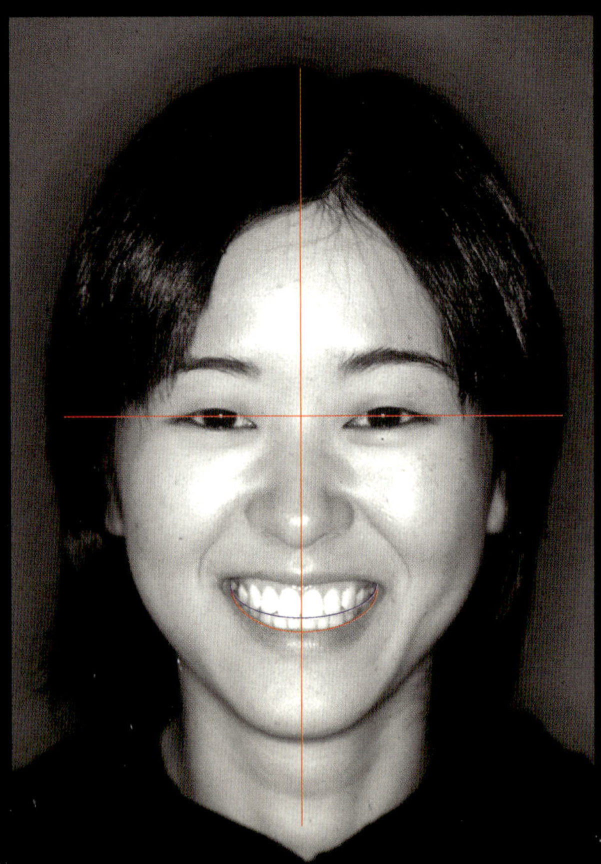

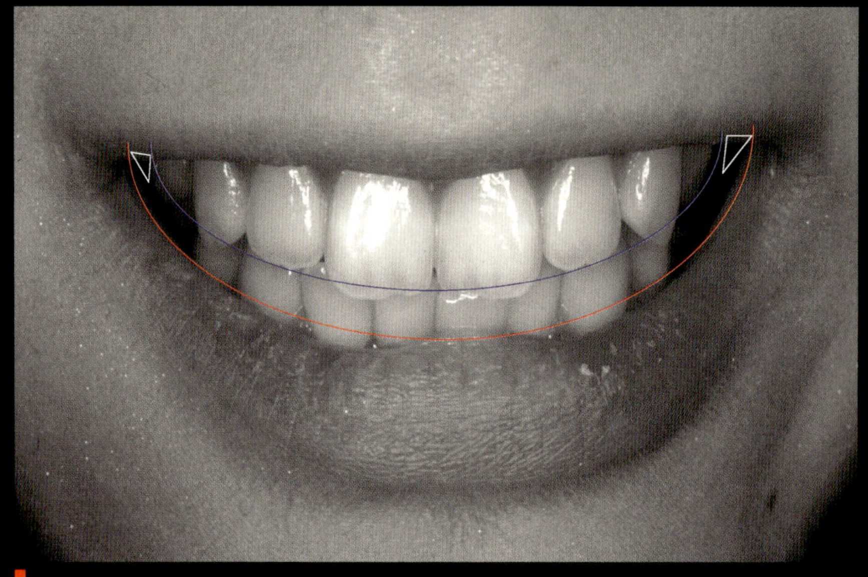

Adult female who has never had dental treatment

An appearance that creates a healthy and appealing impression largely corresponds to the objective criteria of esthetics. The term "buccal corridor" refers to the dark triangles between the corners of the mouth and the teeth (white triangles in figure). The buccal corridor is an esthetically important factor because it gives the row of teeth a three-dimensional appearance and adds charm to the smile.

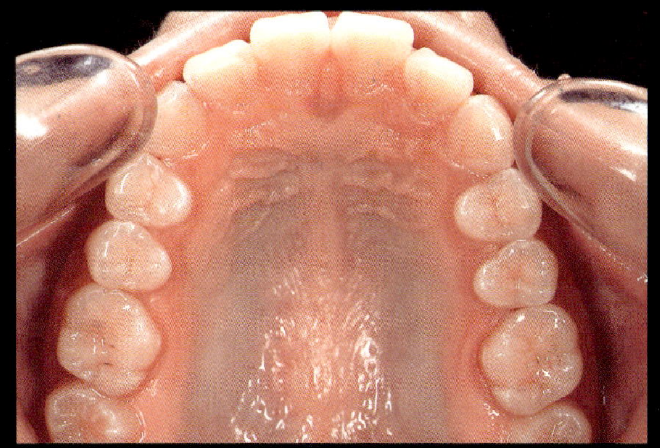

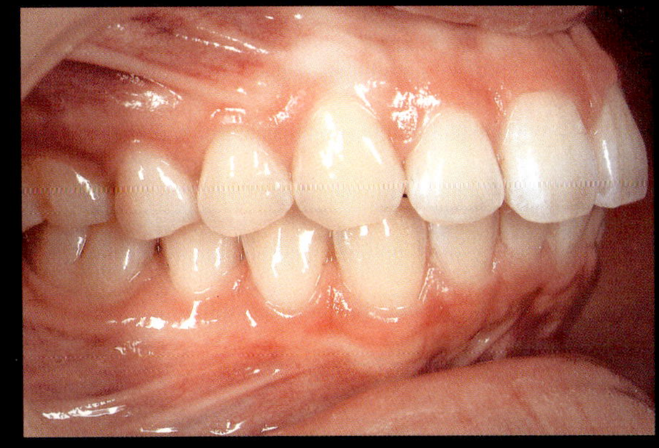

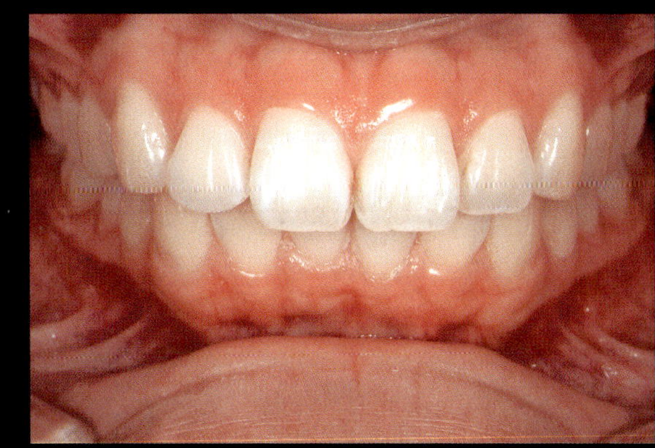

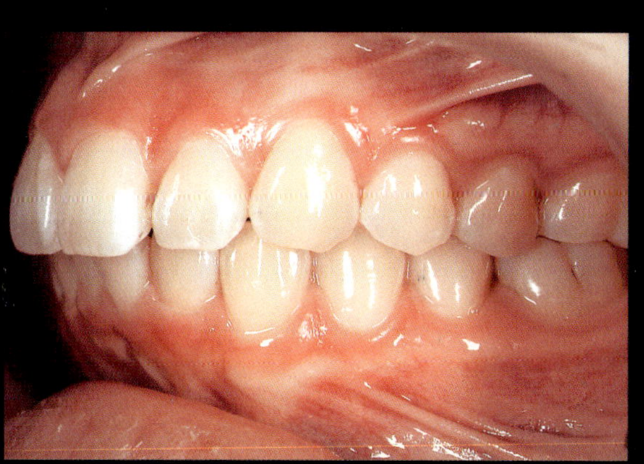

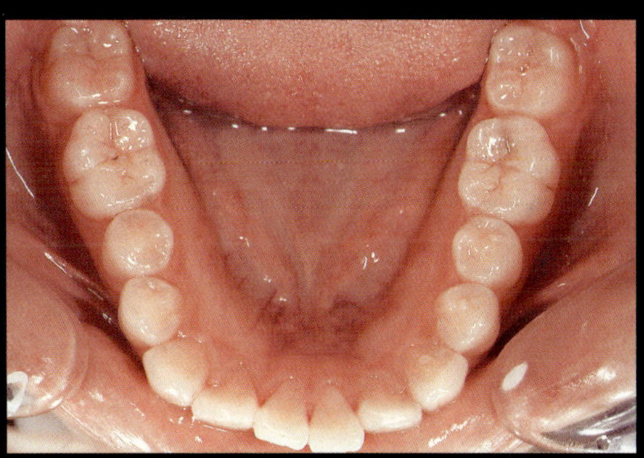

Fully intact dentition

Intact individual teeth and rows of teeth largely fulfill the objective criteria of esthetics.

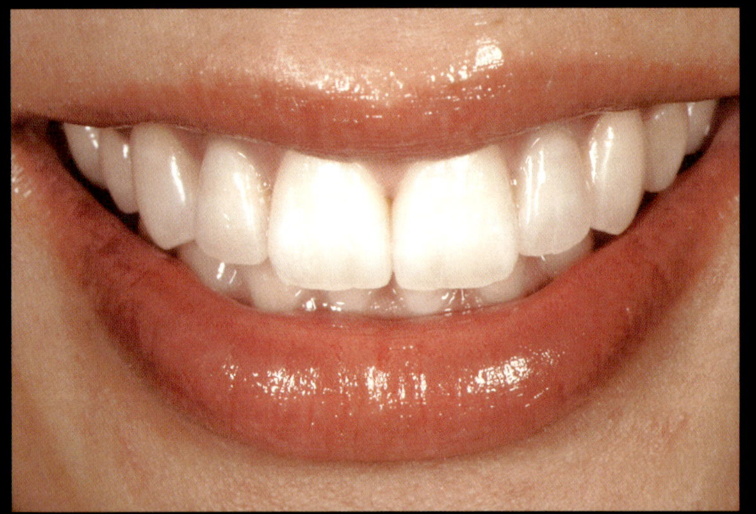

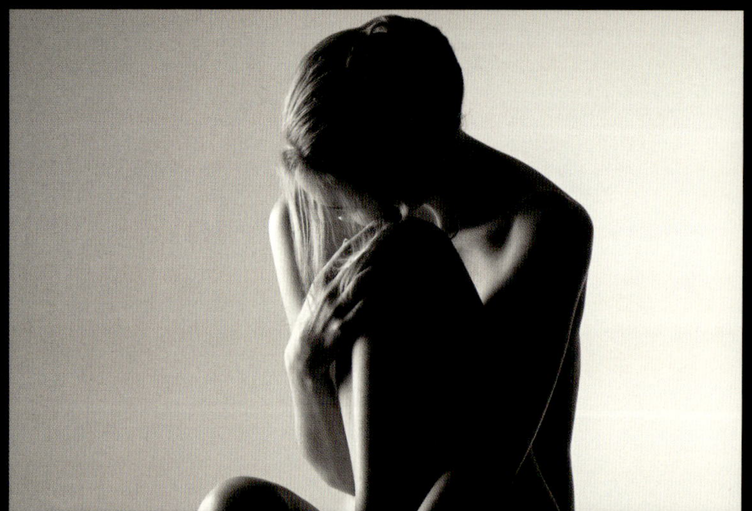

Feminine

A feminine smile is characterized by a bow-shaped lower lip that extends parallel to the incisal line of the upper lip. Women generally have a high smile line.

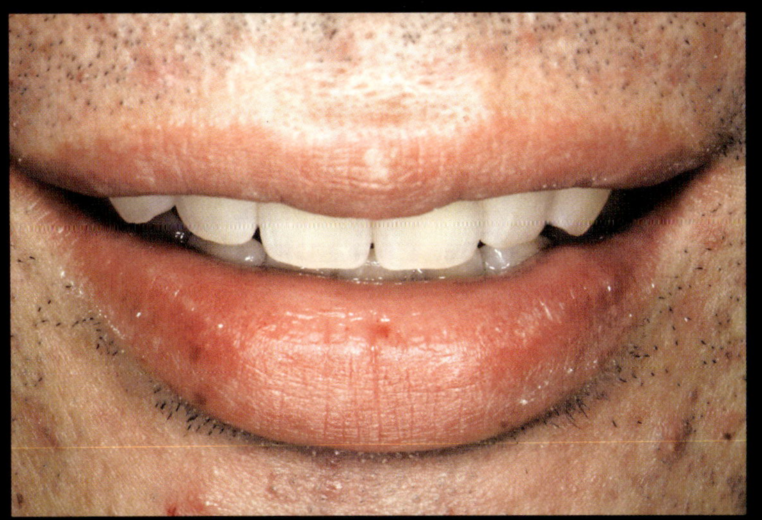

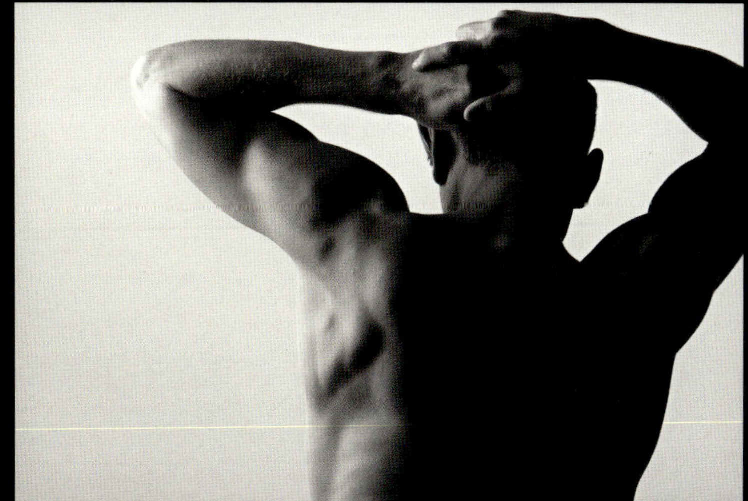

Masculine

A masculine smile is characterized by a straight incisal line that conveys the impression of health and strength. Men generally have a low smile line.

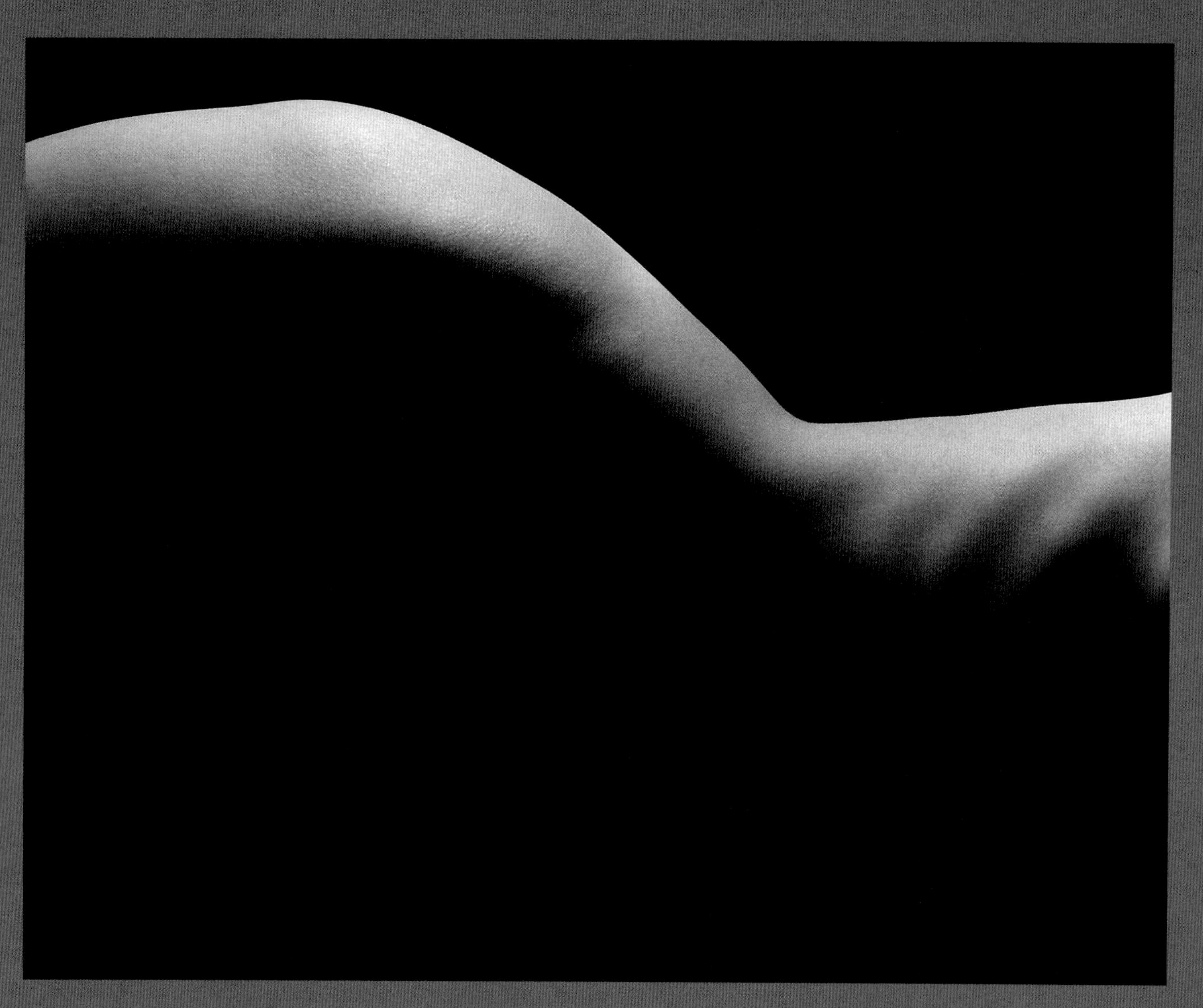

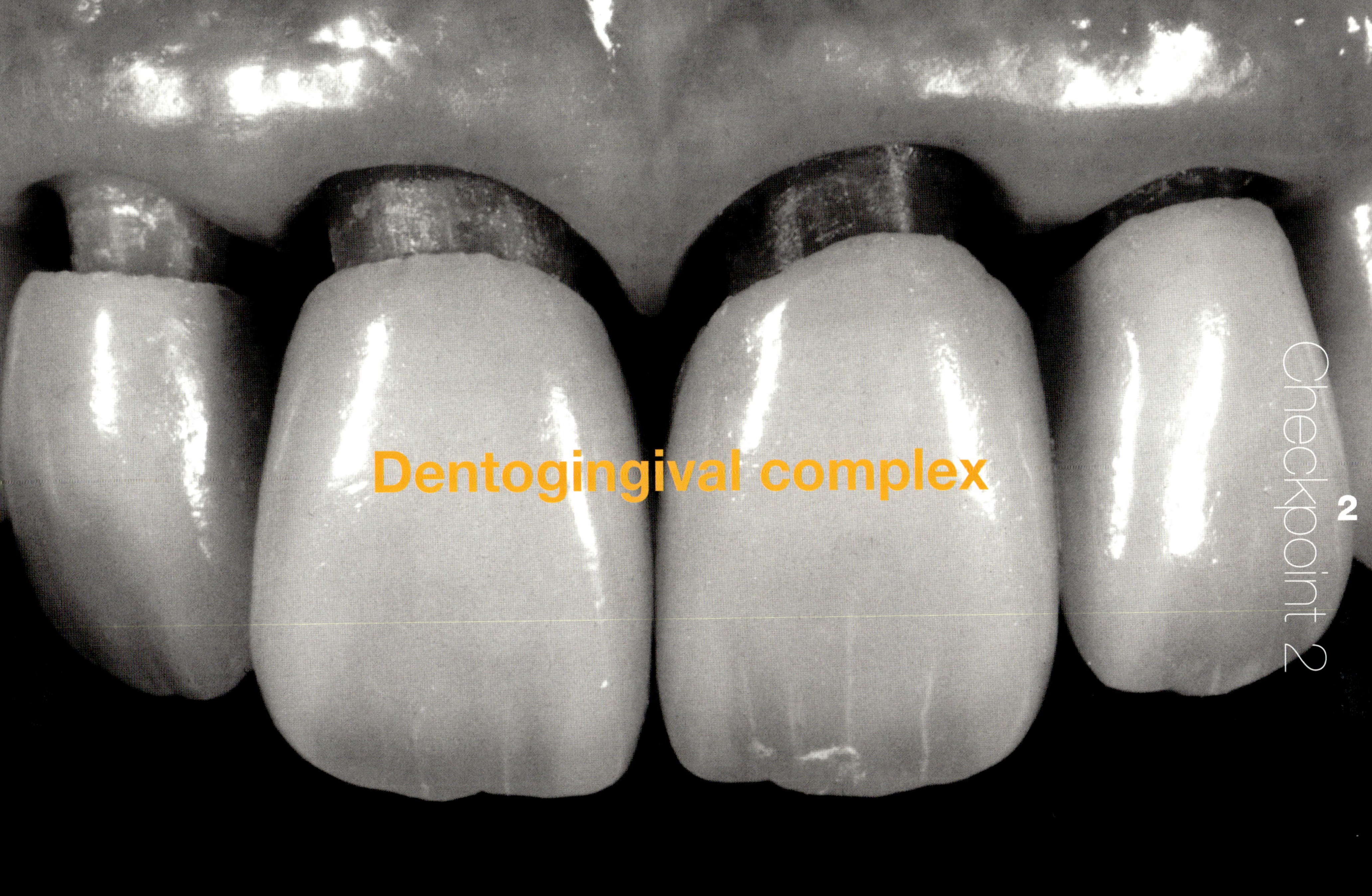

Checkpoint 2

Dentogingival complex

Anatomy of the teeth and periodontium: In order to perform restorative dentistry, one must have a profound knowledge of the anatomy of the teeth and their attachment apparatus.

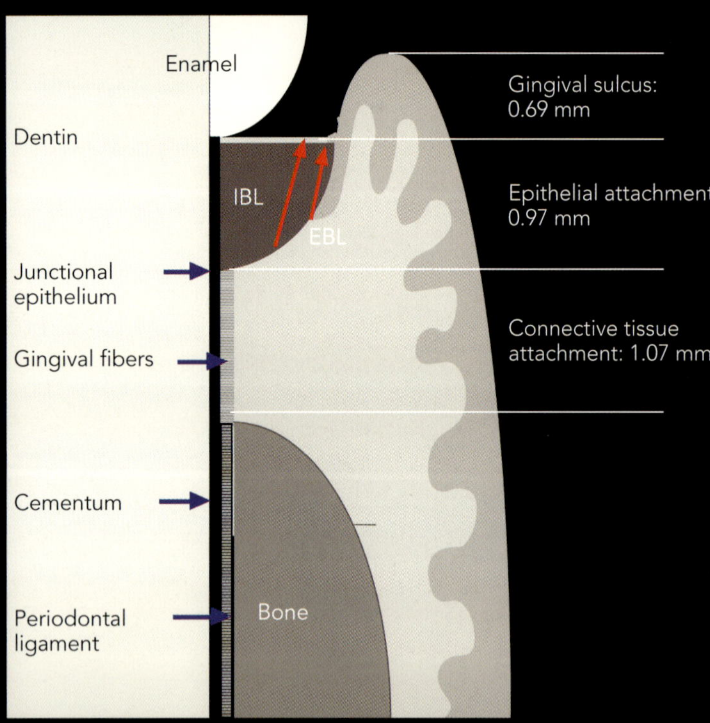

Biologic width

Gargiulo 1961

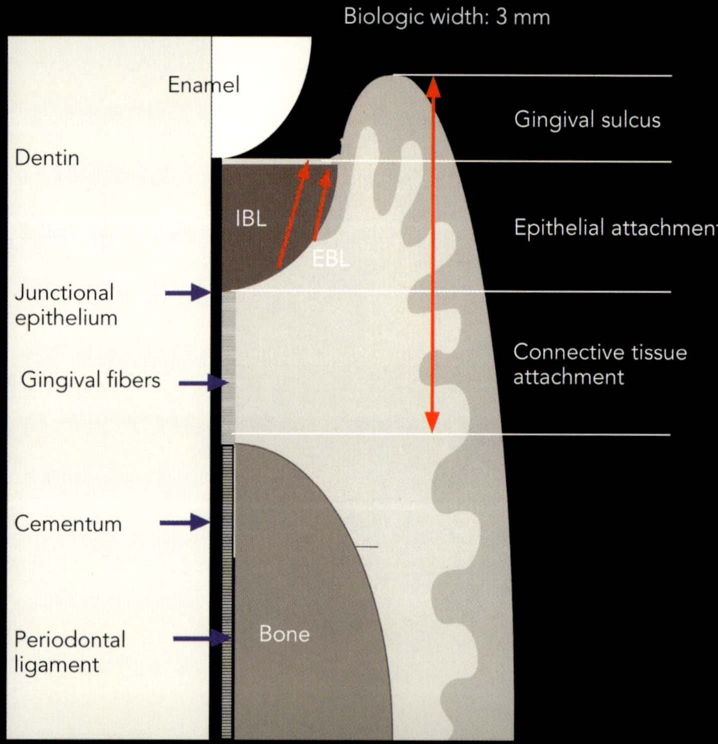

Biologic width

Nevins 1984

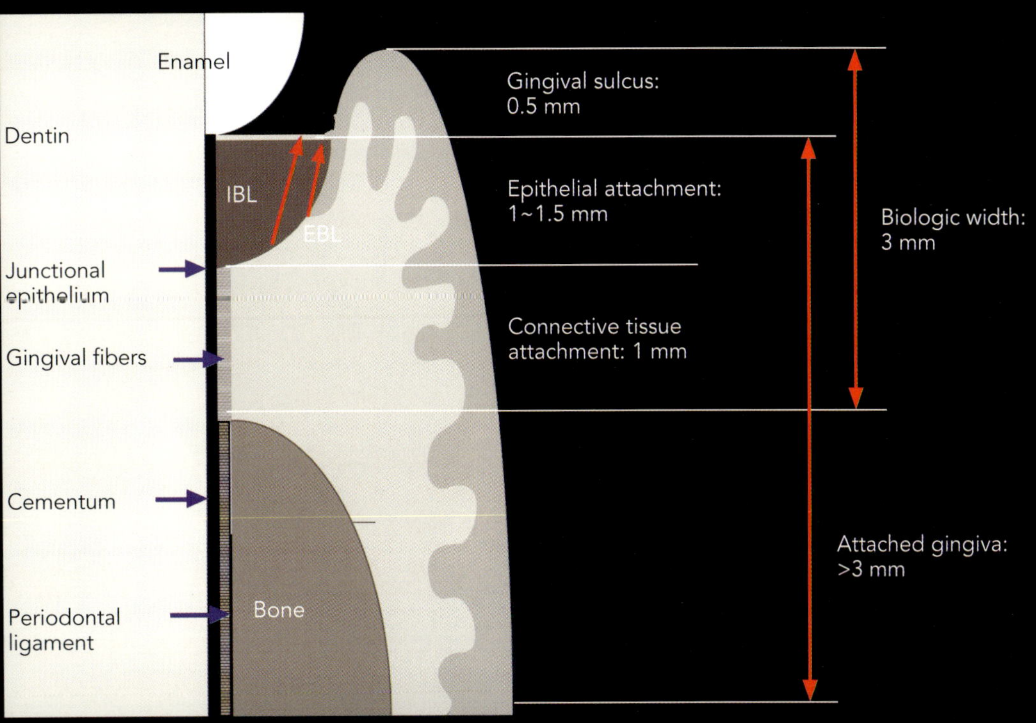

Tooth-periodontium relationships

Biologic width (p. 12)

Gargiulo et al. (1961) reported the following dimensions: gingival sulcus depth: 0.69 mm (0.00–5.36 mm), epithelial attachment width: 0.97 mm (0.16–3.72 mm) and connective tissue attachment width: 1.07 mm (0.00–6.52 mm). These data are based on the study of 287 teeth from cadavers (age at time of death: 19–50 years).

Nevins et al. (1984) observed that the combined dimension of the gingival sulcus and connective tissue attachments (attached gingiva) is approximately 3 mm. They defined this dimension at the individual tooth surfaces as the *biologic width*. In order to maintain the structure of the periodontium, the body responds to changes by initiating resorption or tissue building processes.

Tooth-periodontium relationships (p. 13)

In the clinical experience of the author, the average sulcus depth in Asian subjects is roughly 0.5 mm. If a subgingival crown margin is planned, the margin will therefore lie about 0.5 mm below the gingival margin.

Attached gingiva (p. 13)

It has been reported that the presence of attached gingiva around a teeth is not essential for tooth survival. However, it is easier to maintain periodontal health when more than 3 mm of keratinized gingiva is present. This applies in particular to restored teeth.

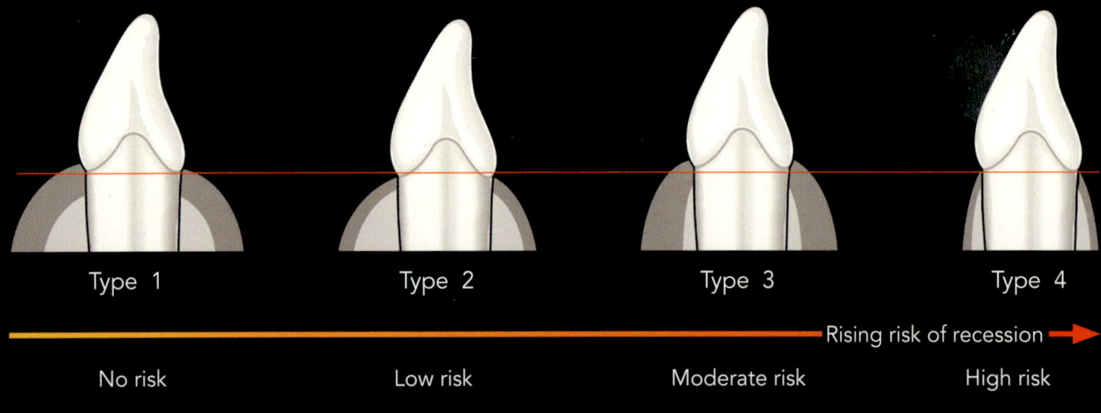

Physiological dimensions of the periodontium

Maynard divided the periodontium into four types according to hard and soft tissue thicknesses. In the opinion of the author, subgingival margin placement of restorations is contraindicated in type 4 (hard and soft tissue).
Biotypes with a thicker periodontium have higher gingival margins.

Biological variants

Kois divided the periodontium into three types according to the height of the alveolar crest. In patients with a high crest, subgingival placement of crown margins should be avoided due to the high risk of gingival recession.

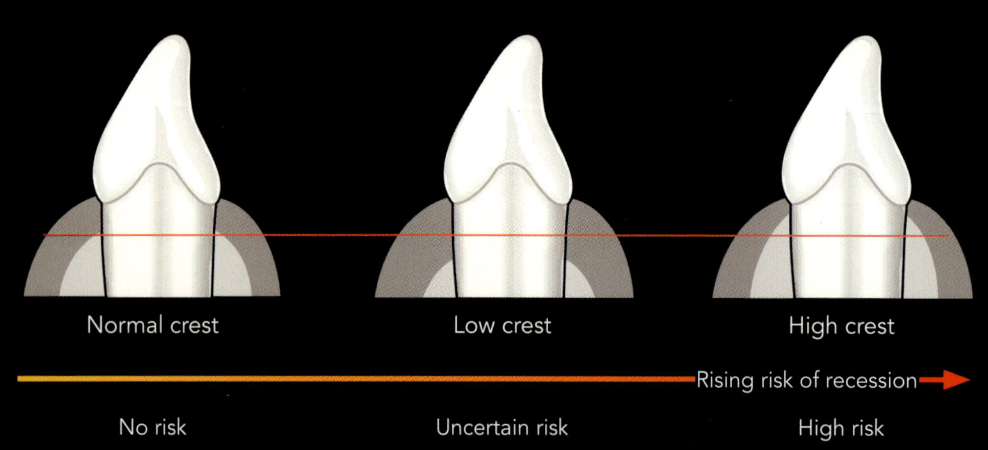

The type of restoration and the position of the crown margin can only be determined after the periodontal situation of the tooth that is to be restored has been analyzed.

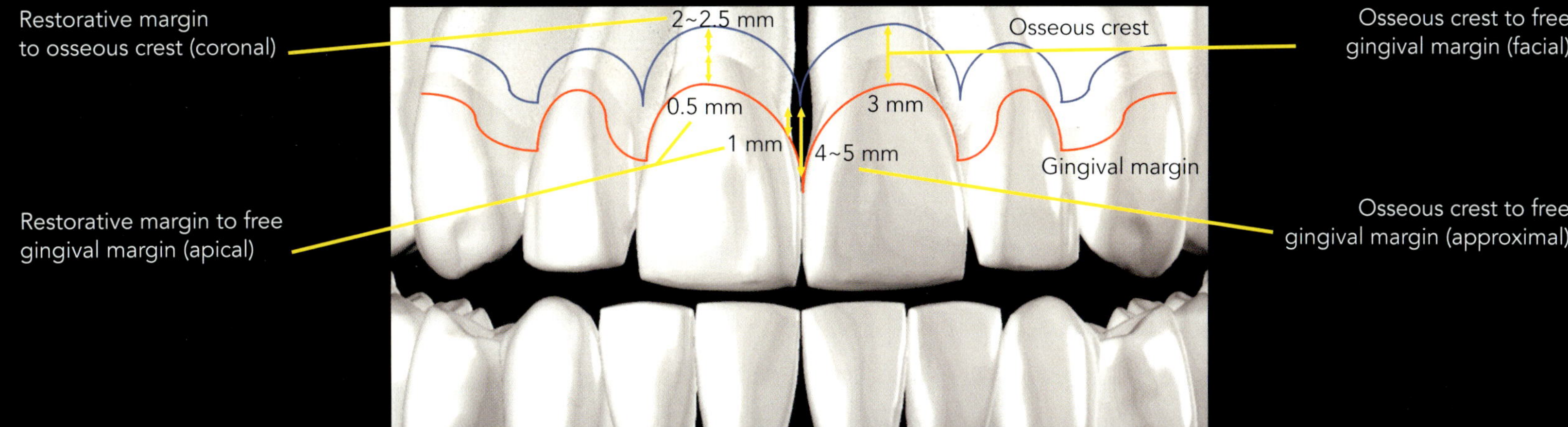

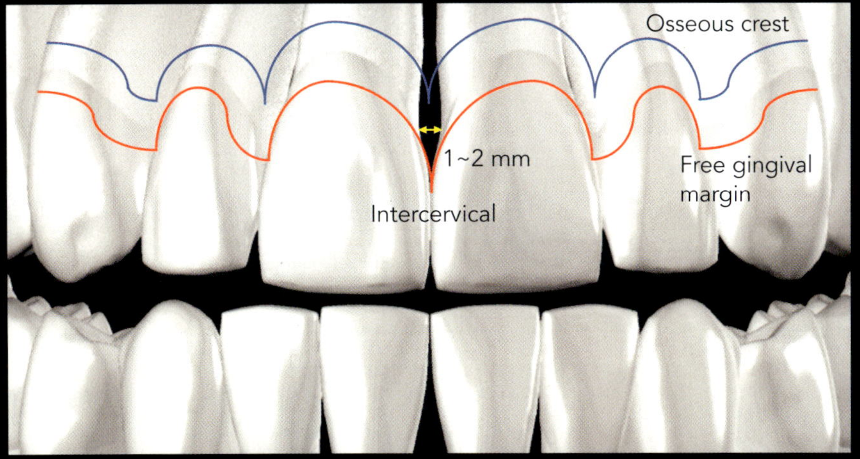

Clinical criteria for esthetic gingival relationships

If the crown margin must be situated subgingivally, it can generally be placed labially up to 0.5 mm below the gingival margin and 2–2.5 mm above the alveolar bone and, approximally, 1 mm below the gingival margin and 2 mm above the alveolar margin. In addition, the height of the approximal contact points should be positioned 4–5 mm above the alveolar bone because the interdental spaces are filled with soft tissue. In order to achieve an esthetically acceptable restoration according to these criteria, the cervical distance between the adjacent abutment teeth must be 1–2 mm.

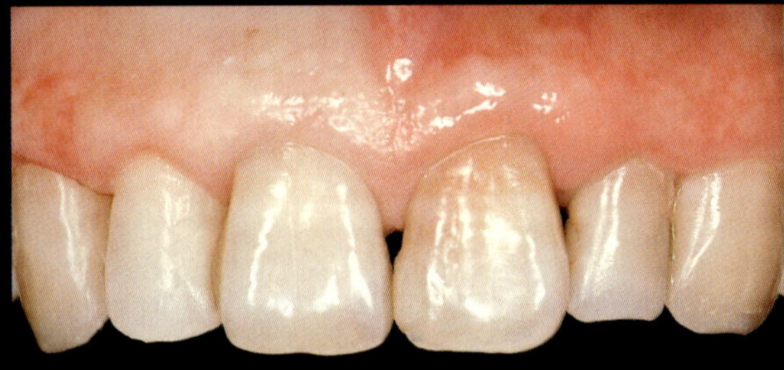

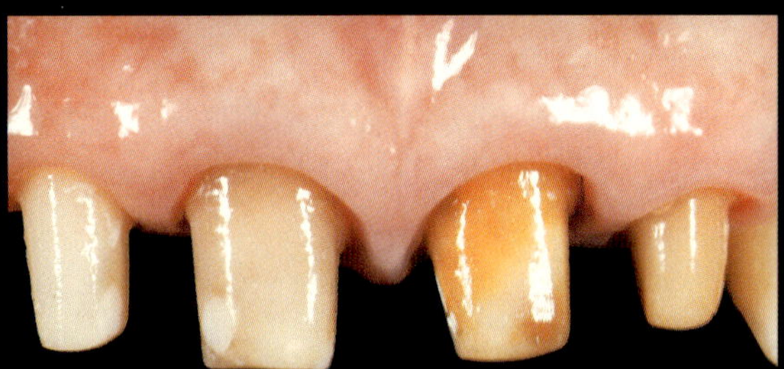

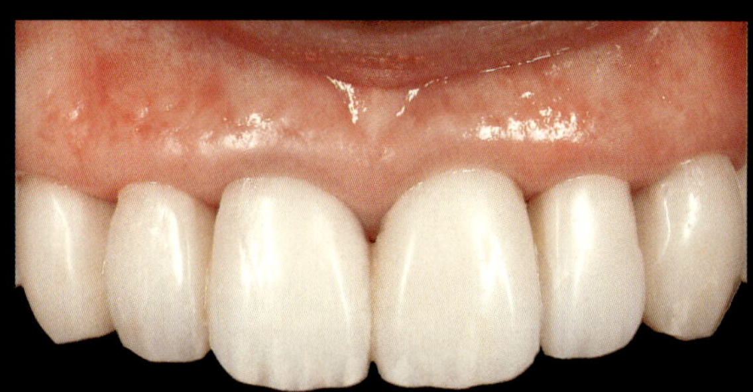

Temporary restoration

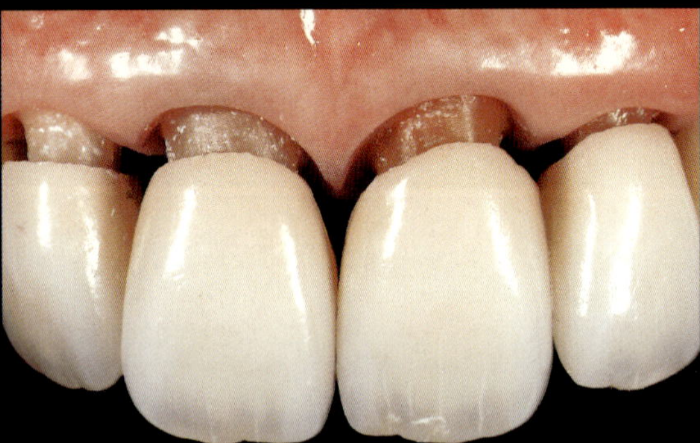

Permanent restoration

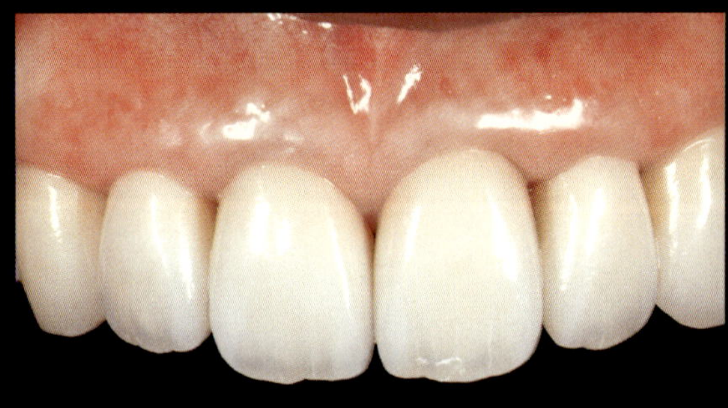

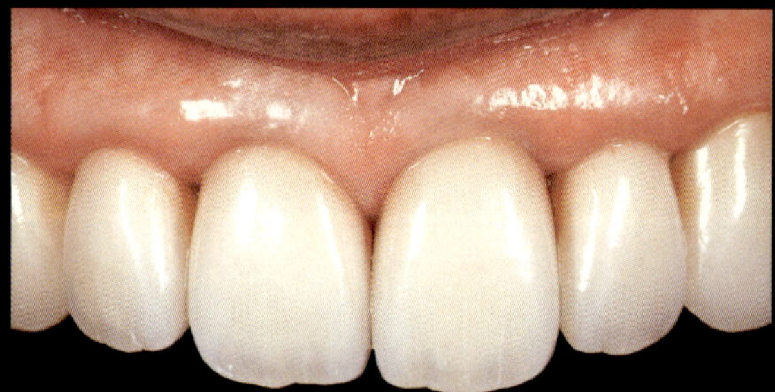

10 years later

Case study

In clinical practice, temporary restorations are planned and placed according to the criteria described above. Permanent restorations are fabricated after small corrections have been made as needed over the course of follow-up.

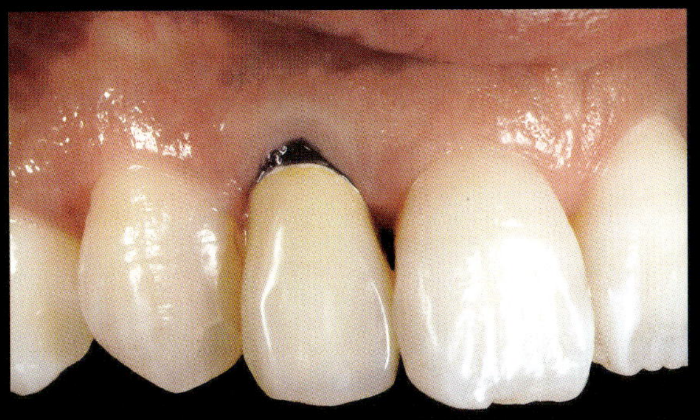
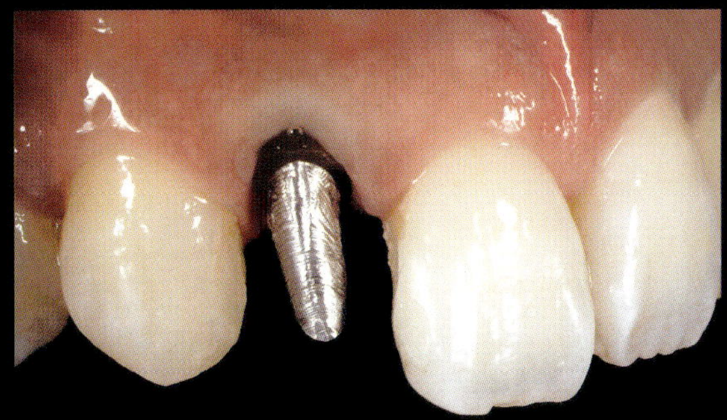
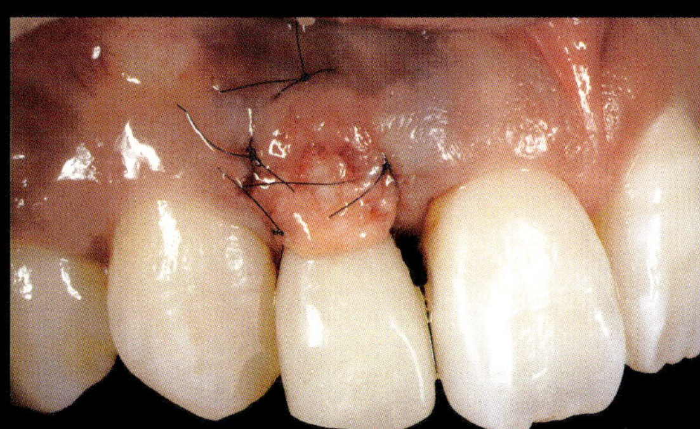
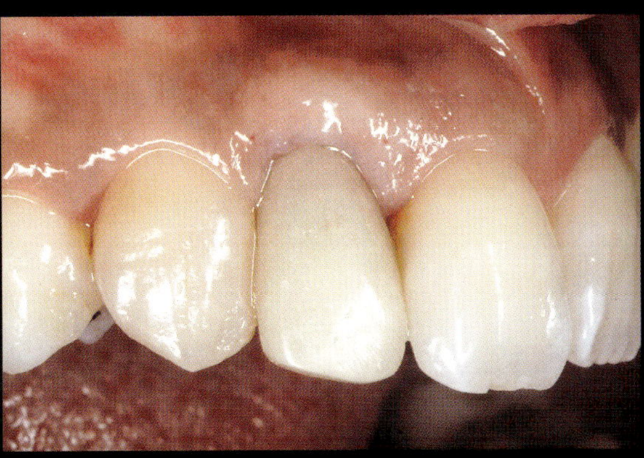
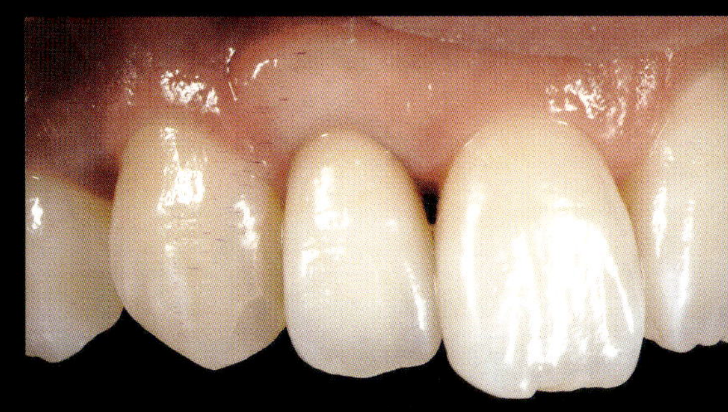

Permanent restoration

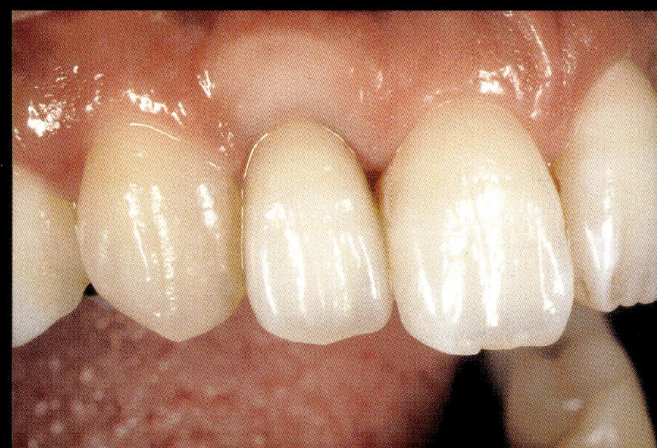

5 years later

Preparation of the surrounding periodontium

According to the studies by Wennström, the relationship between gingival height and width tends to be 1 to 1.5. When gingivoplasty is performed, this knowledge can be applied to create more stable periodontal conditions. One can then transform a Maynard type 2 periodontium into a type 1 situation or a Maynard type 4 periodontium into a type 3, or transform an alveolar crest that is high according to the Kois classification into a normal crest.

In the case shown here, a connective tissue graft was used to close the exposed discolored root surface and to increase the volume of the soft tissue layer.

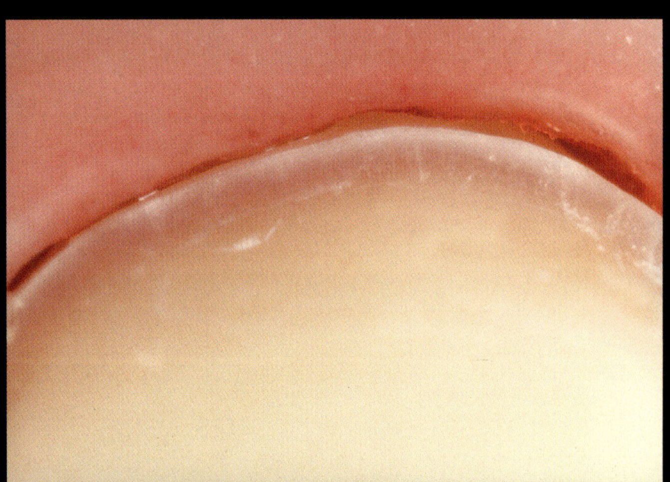

Magnified preparation margin

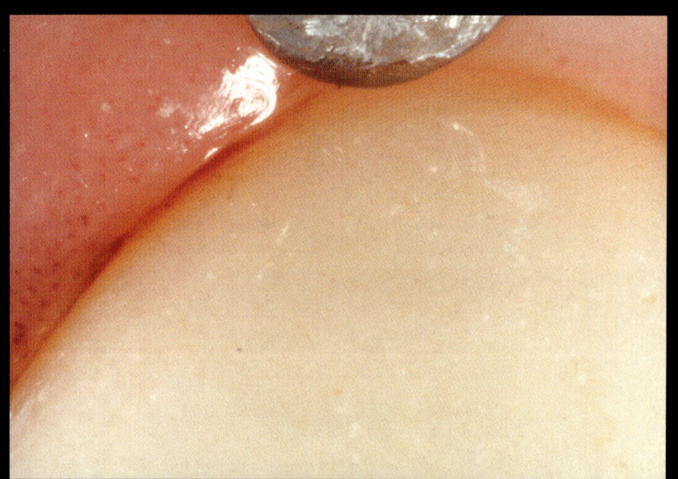

Adapted preparation margin

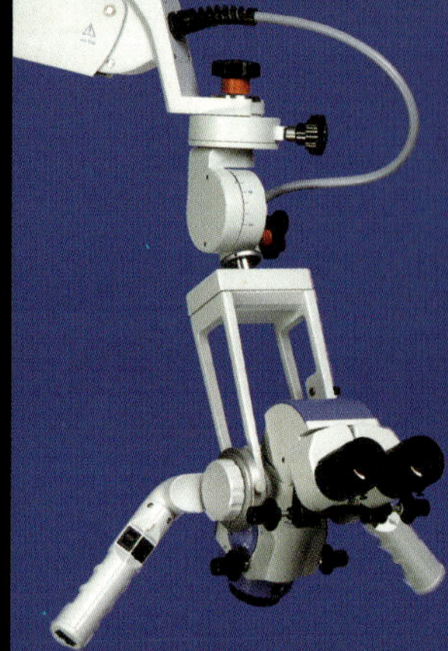

Enhanced precision through magnification

With the aid of a stereoscopic microscope, preparation margins can be adapted with high precision for excellent crown fit.

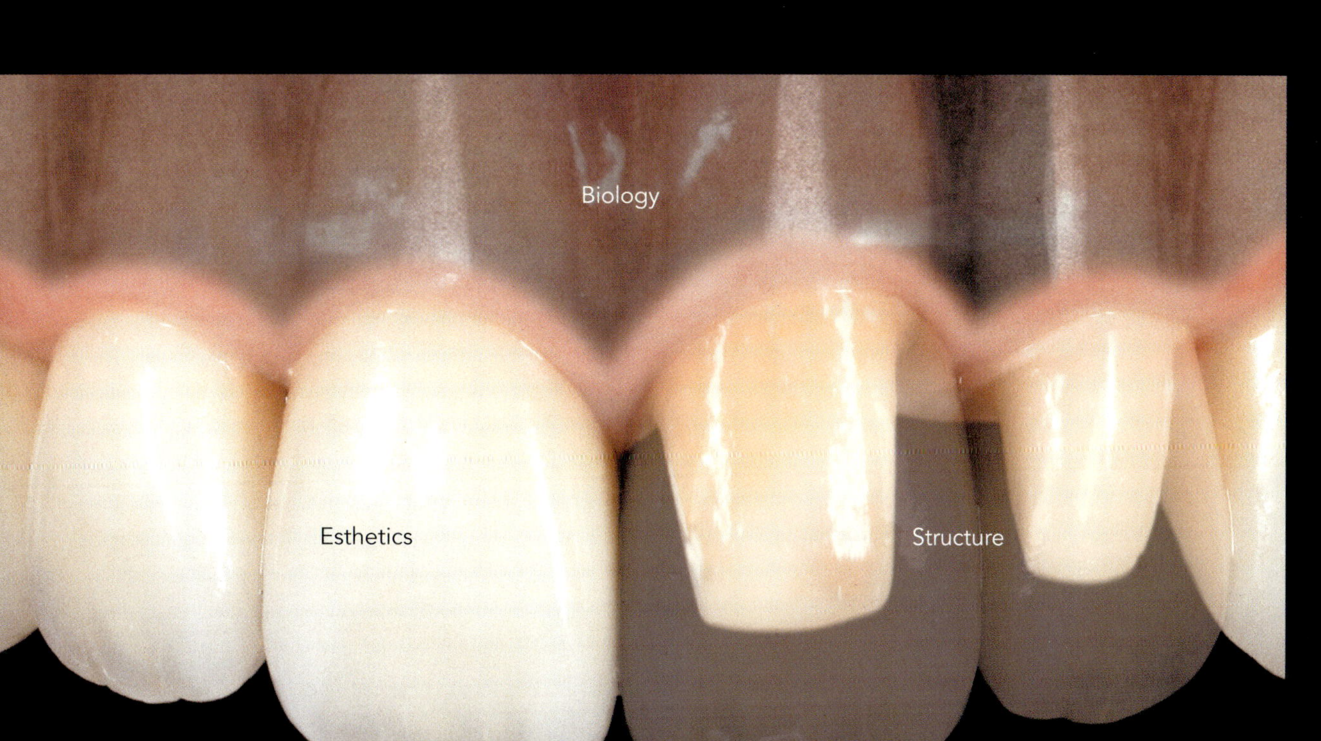
Biology
Esthetics
Structure

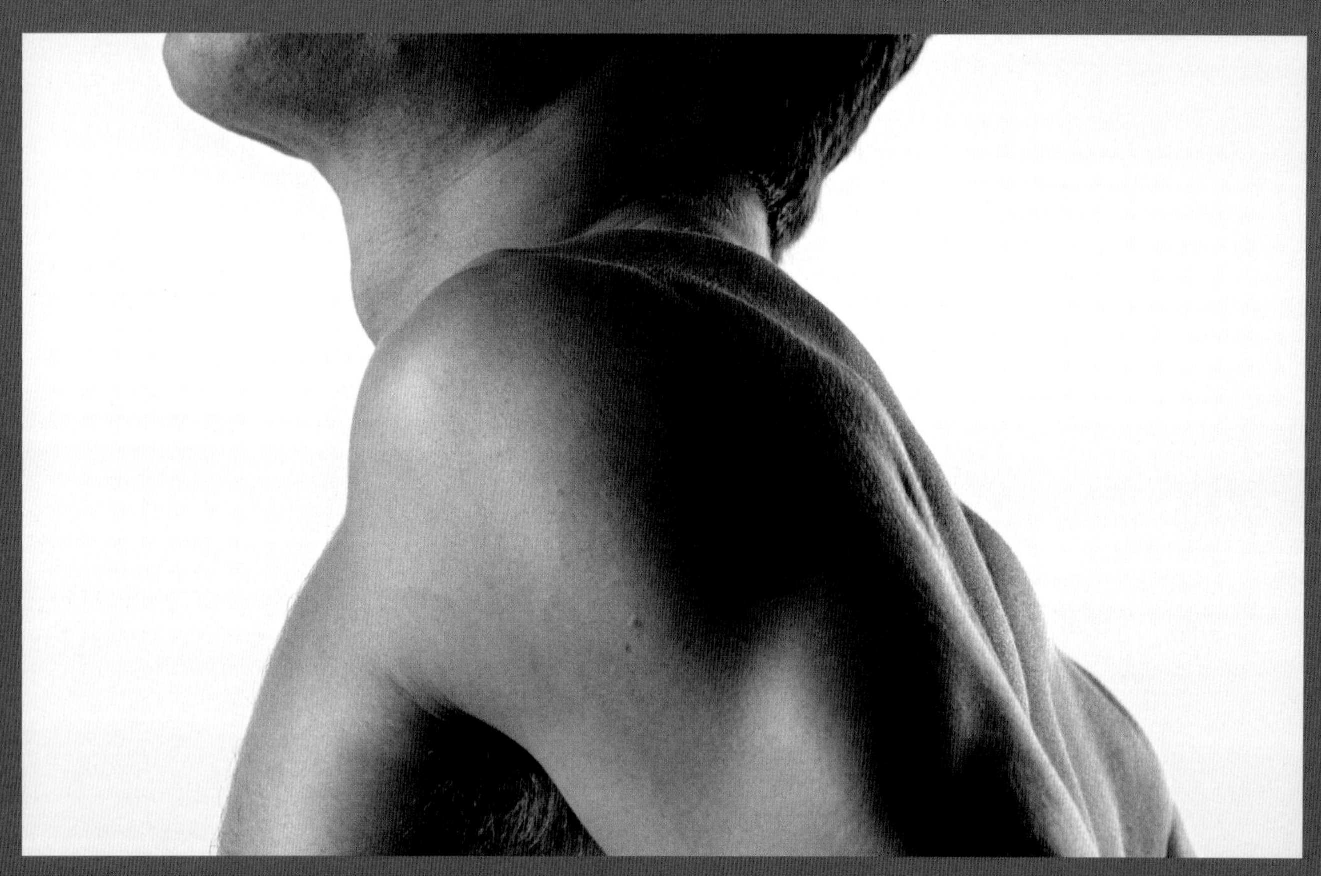

Axial crown contours

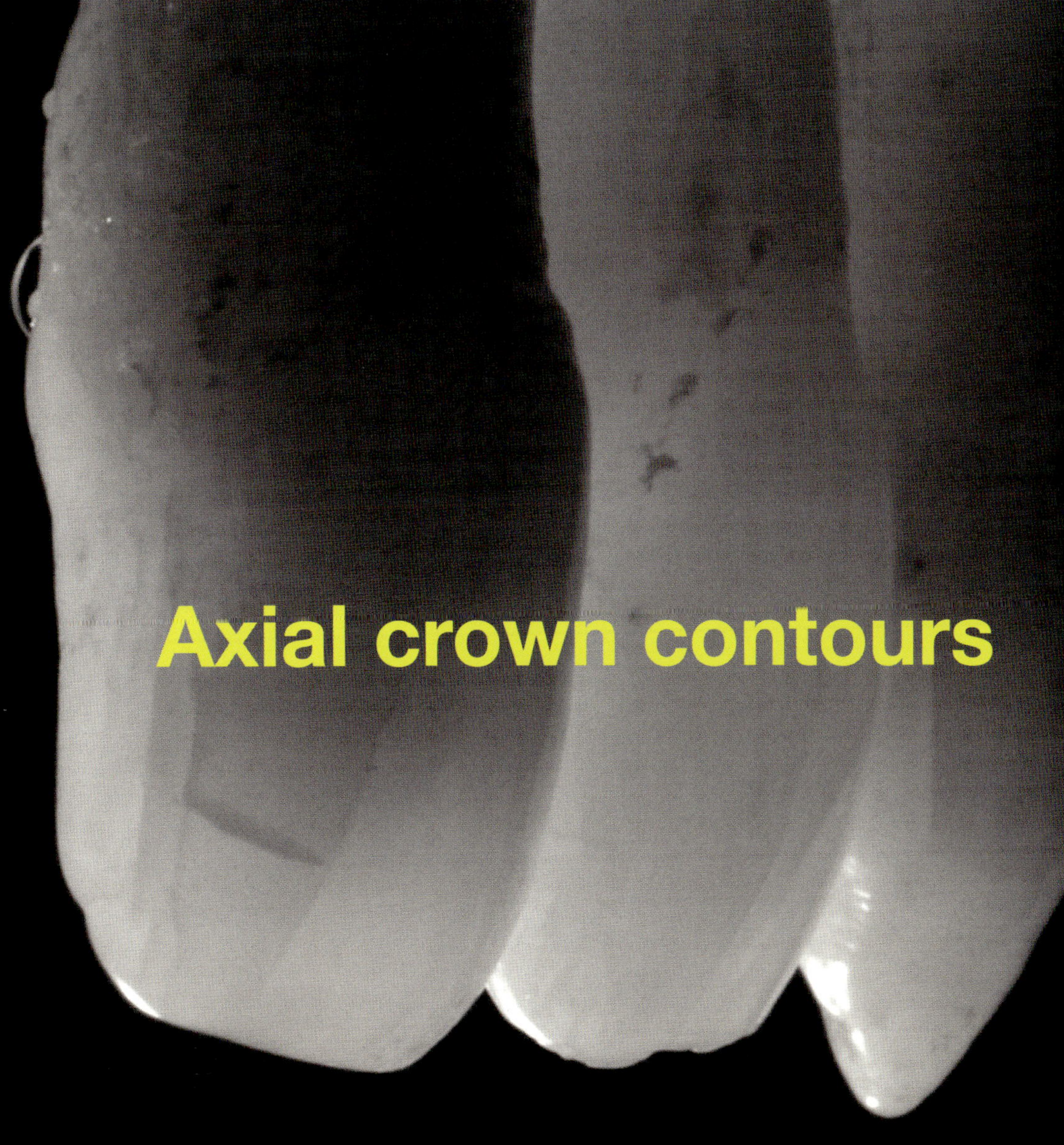

Knowledge of axial tooth contours is essential for successful restorative treatment.
Differences in contour can be seen in the three teeth shown on page 21 (left-right: central incisor, lateral incisor and cuspid).

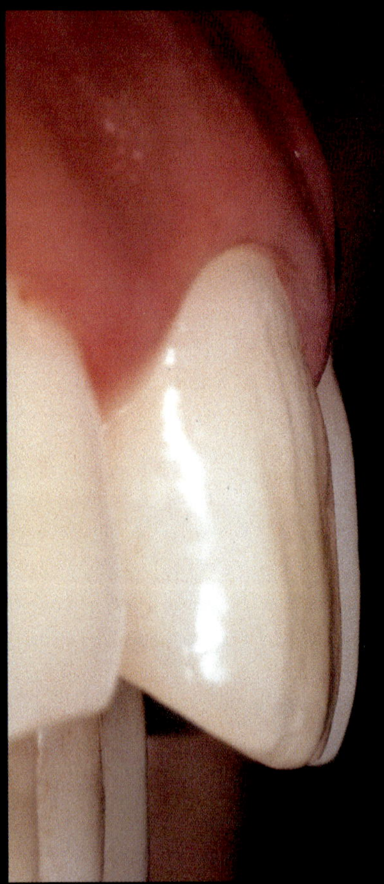

Intact teeth

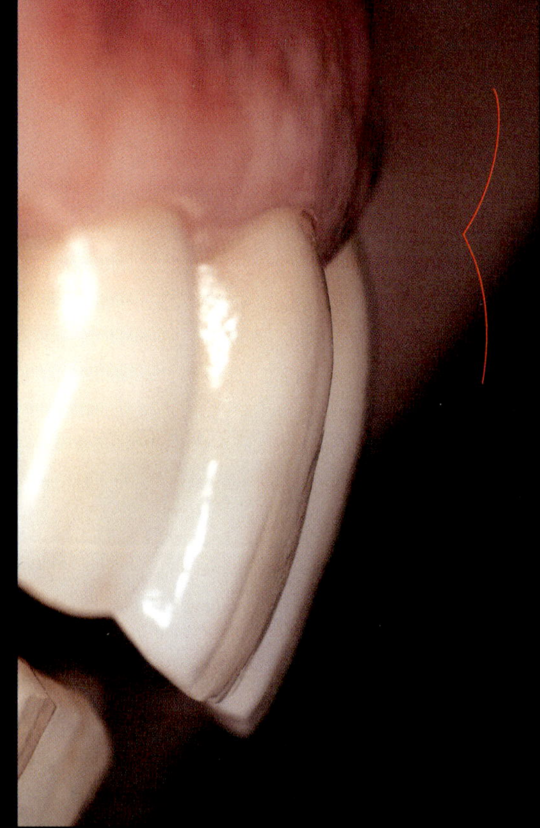

PFM crowns

Axial crown contours (Gull wing)

On inspection of the teeth and periodontium, one can see that the cervical to coronal contour is symmetrical to the apical contour. Dragoo et al. described this symmetry as a "gull wing" pattern. Knowledge of this pattern can be helpful when creating crown contours.

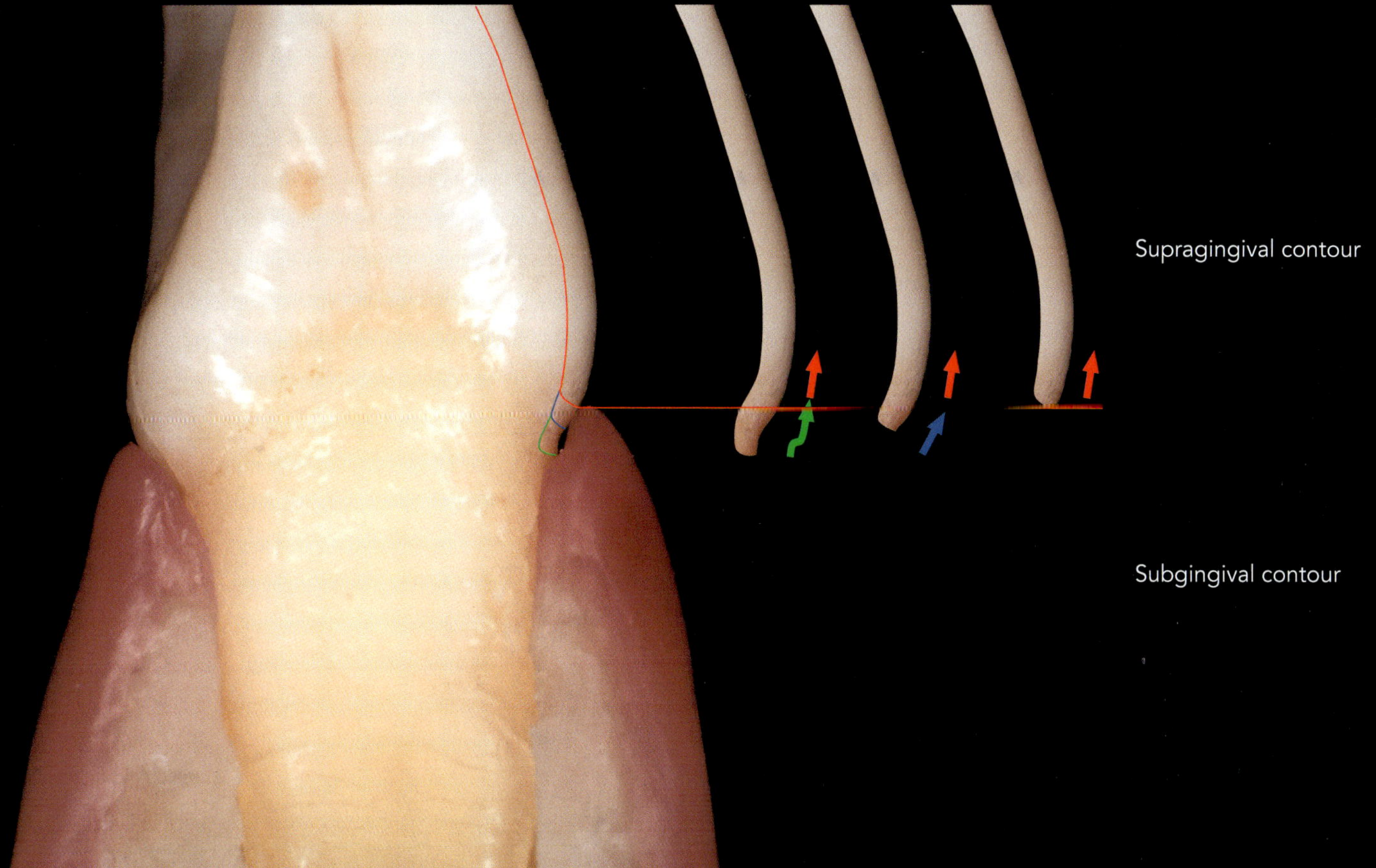

Axial crown contours (Crown margin)

Supragingival and subgingival crown contours must be analyzed separately. The contour of the crown itself can vary depending on the position of the crown, but its supragingival contour always remains the same.

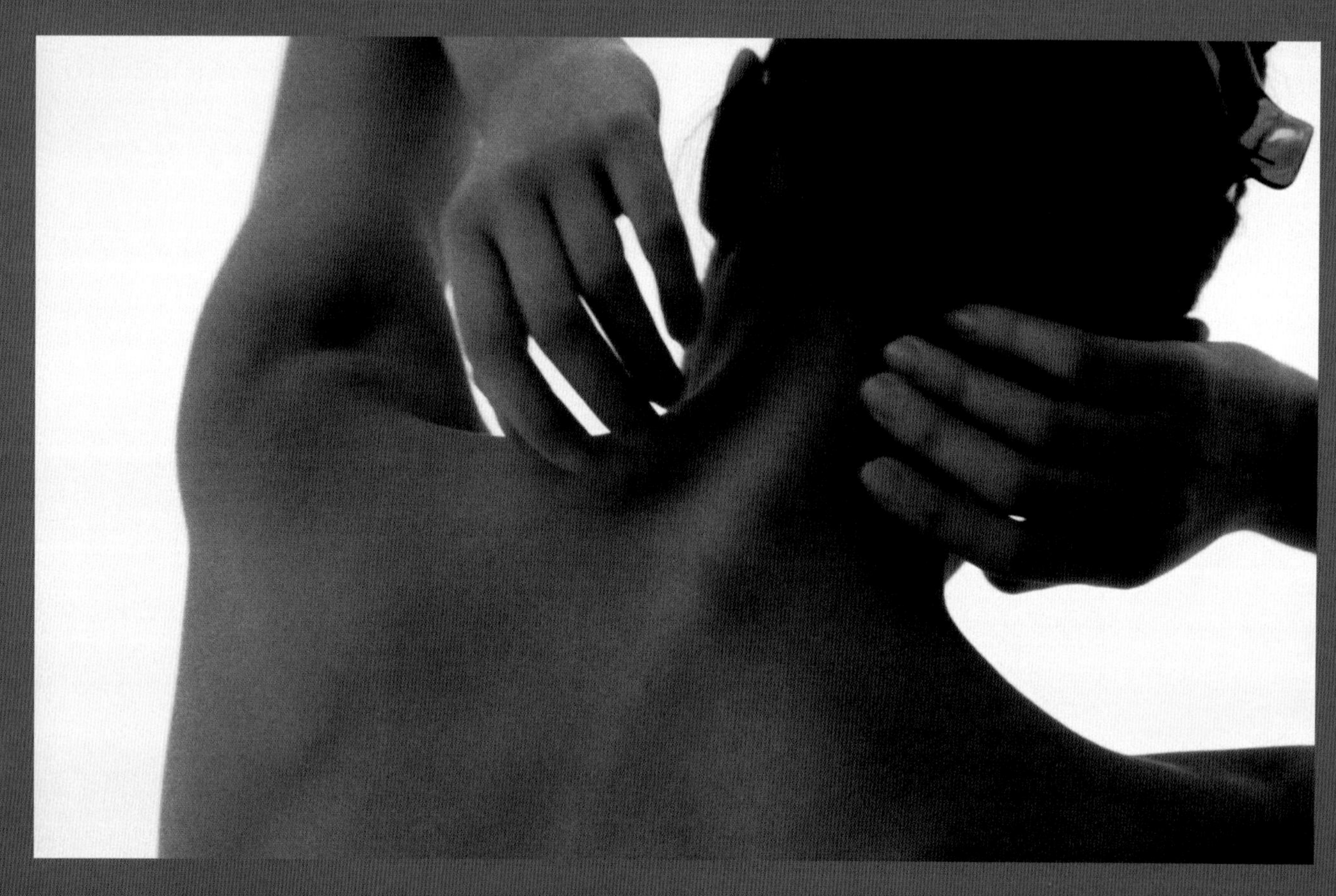

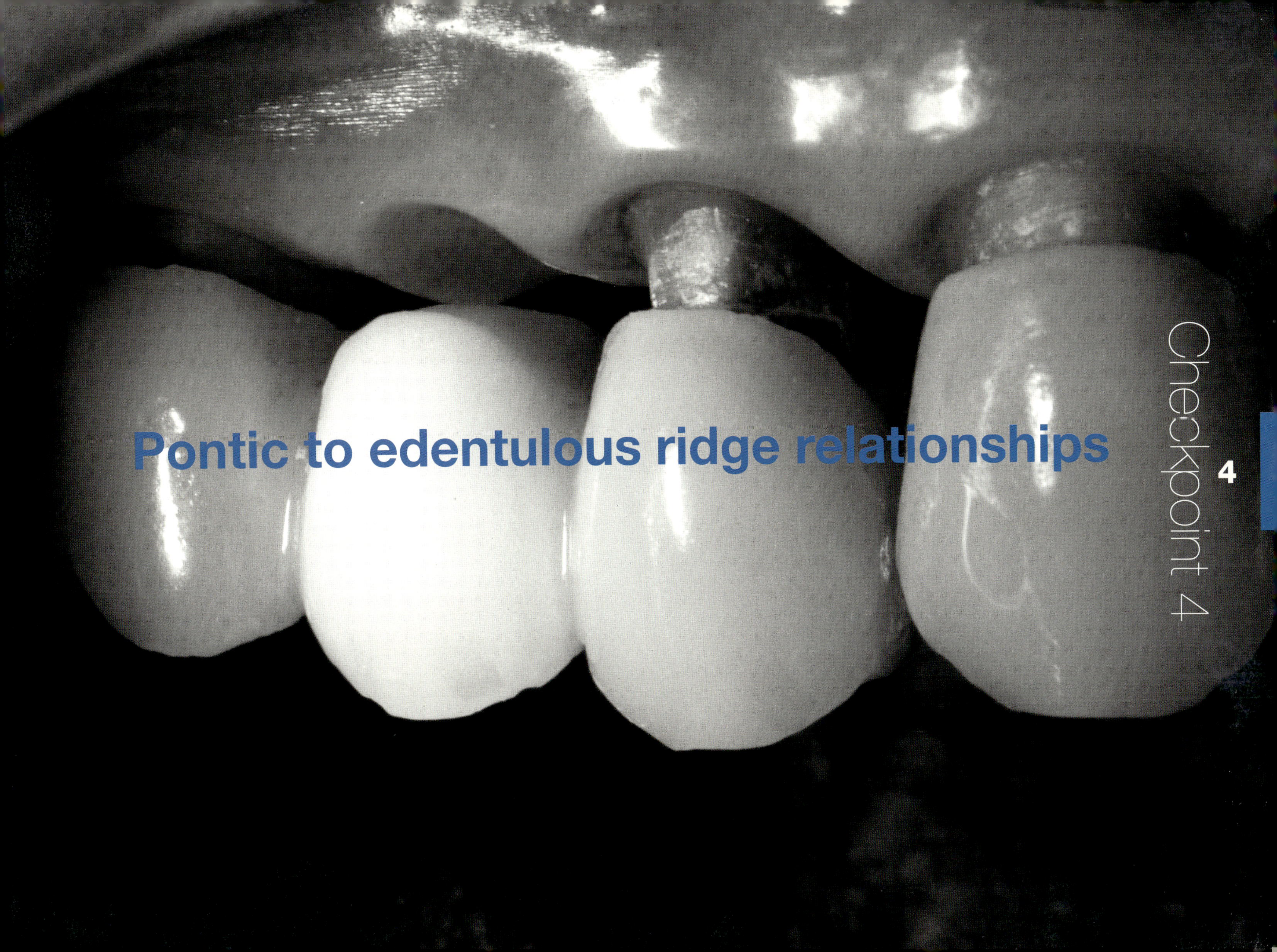

Pontic to edentulous ridge relationships

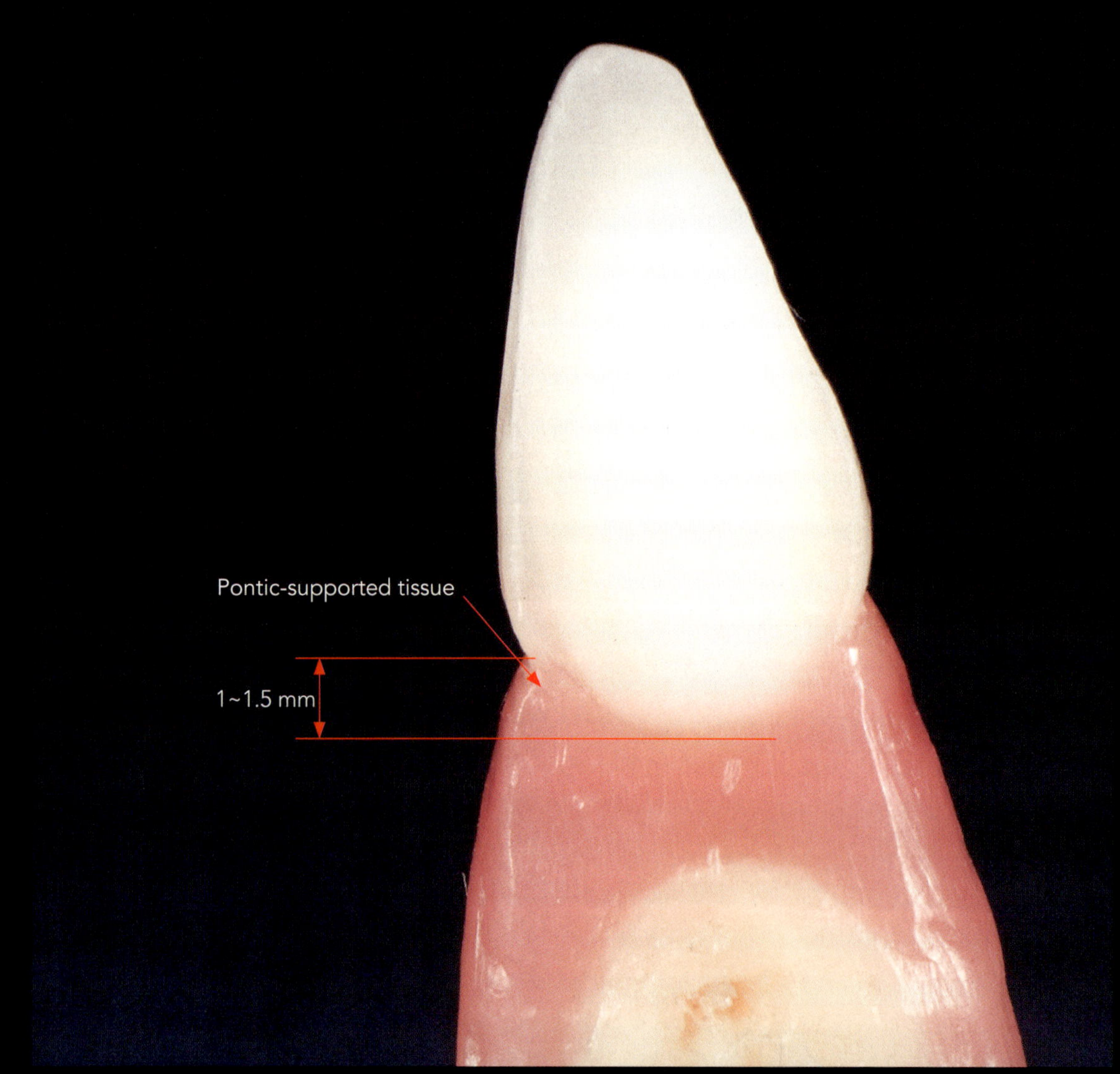

Ovate pontic

Ovate pontics are not only esthetically pleasing but also easy to clean. The pontic recipient site is convex in the buccolingual and mesiodistal direction, and the subgingival depth is 1–1.5 mm. The contours of the pontic slope gently in the coronal direction.

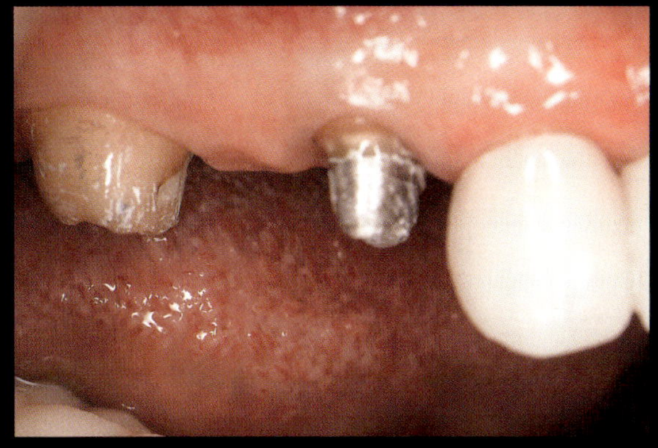

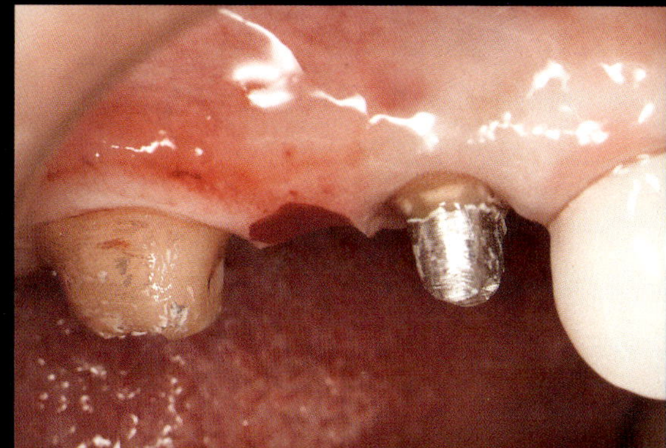

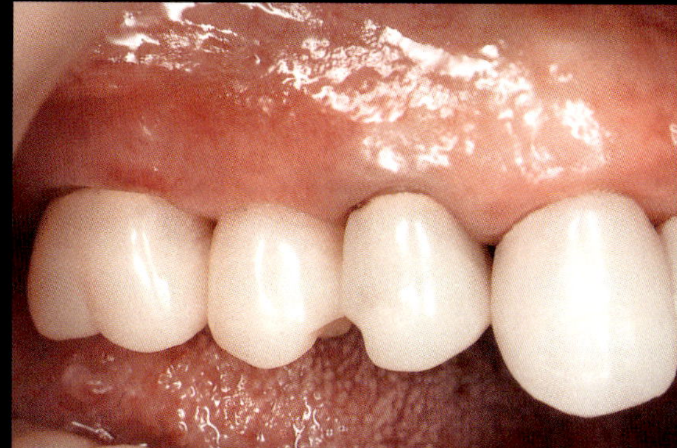

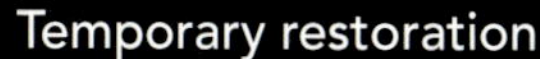

Temporary restoration

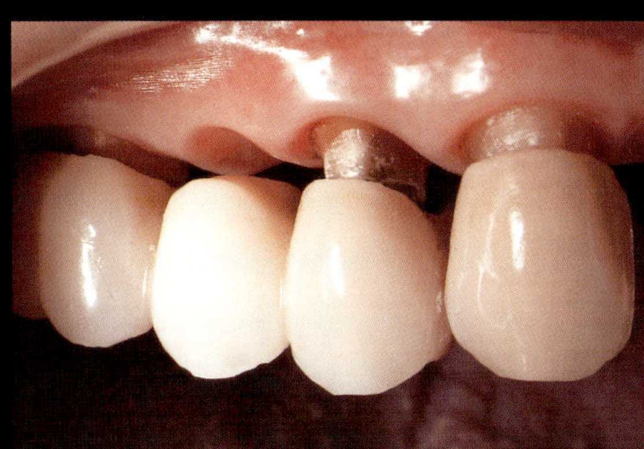

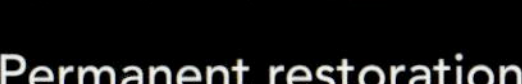

Permanent restoration

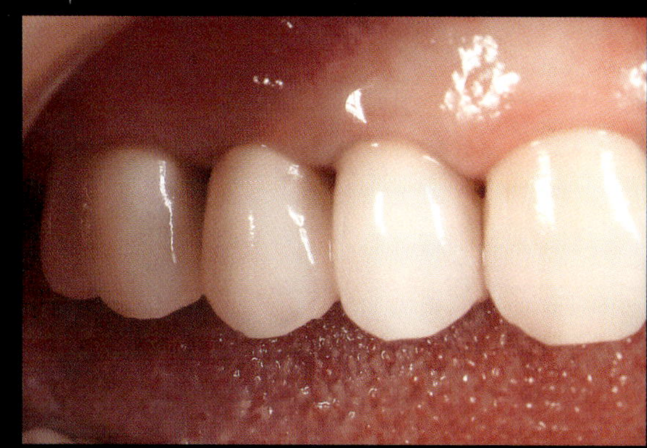

9 years later

Case study 1

After ovate preparation of the edentulous ridge with a diamond instrument, autopolymerizing resin was applied to the basal surface of the temporary pontic, and the pontic was inserted in the prepared concave recipient site. The permanent restoration was placed after allowing the soft tissue to heal completely. Since the base of the ovate pontic was made to fit perfectly in the soft tissue and a pseudo-papilla was formed, there was no detectable infiltration of plaque. This facilitated the cleaning process.

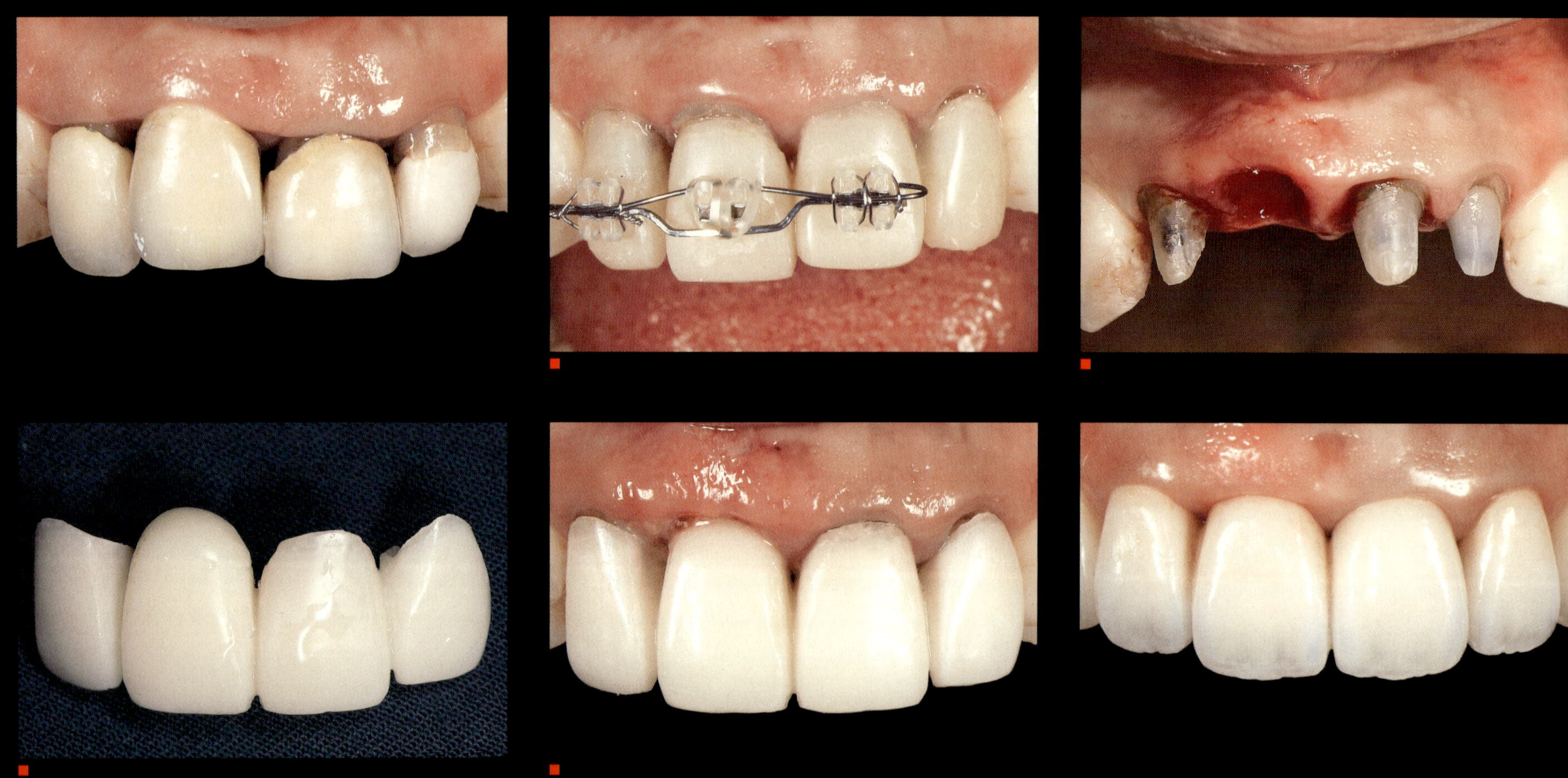

Temporary restoration

5 years later

Case study 2: Immediate loading of an ovate pontic

Controlled tooth extraction is essential for achieving good results. If both hard and soft tissues are present in the extraction wound, a temporary pontic with an oval base should be used. Since approximately 1–2 mm of the surrounding tissue may be absorbed, the base should be placed 2–3 mm subgingivally.

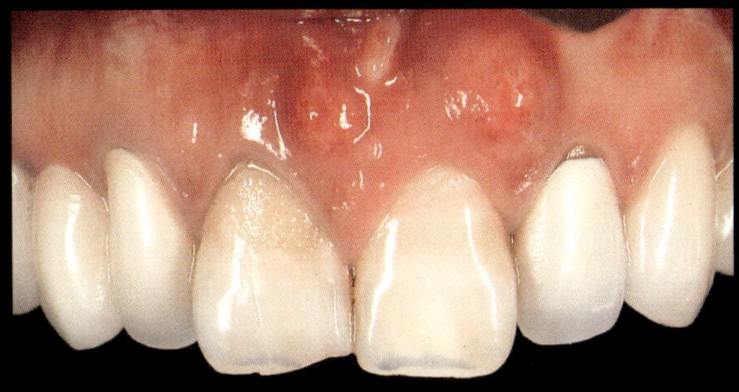

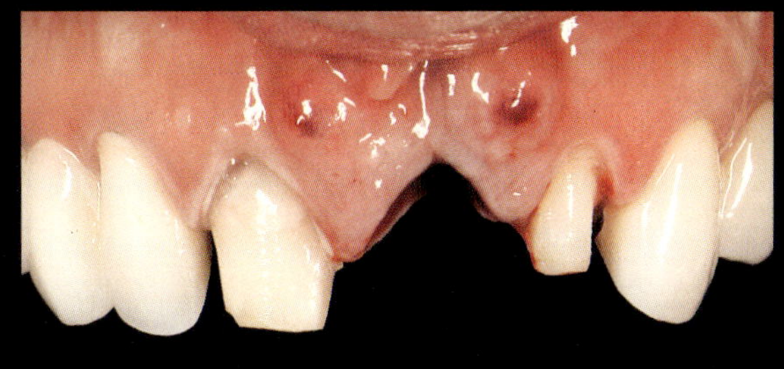

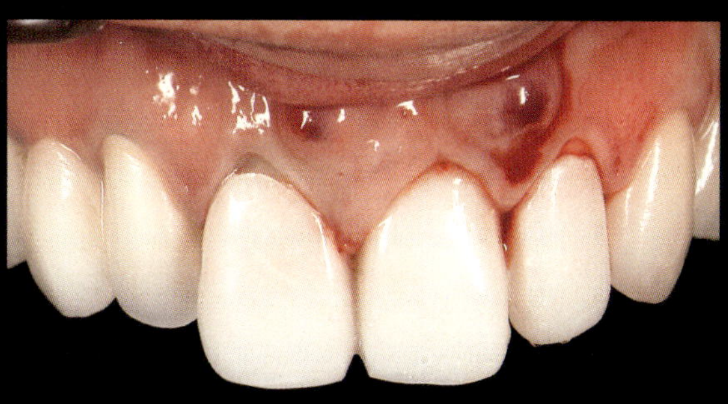

Temporary restoration

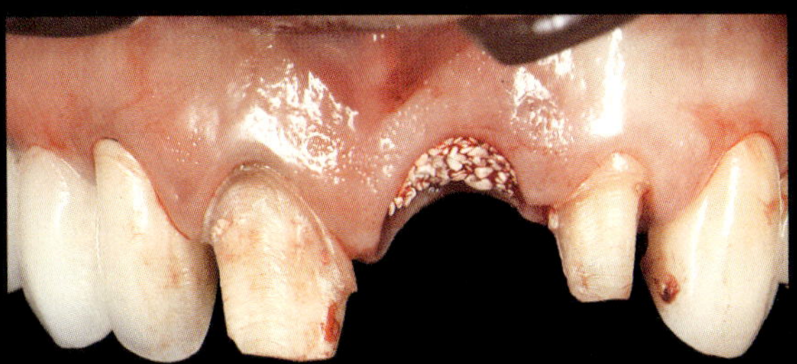

1 week later

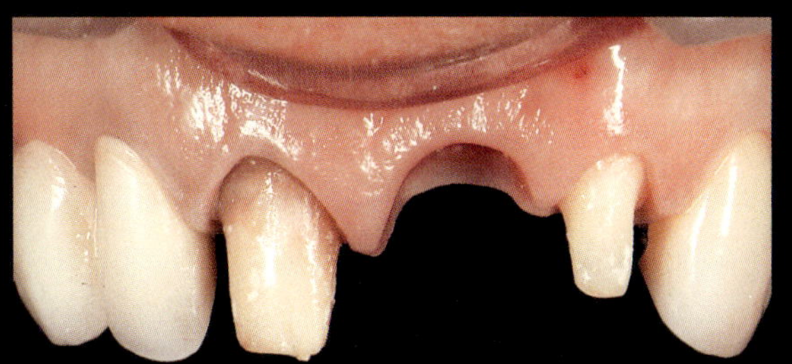

3 months later

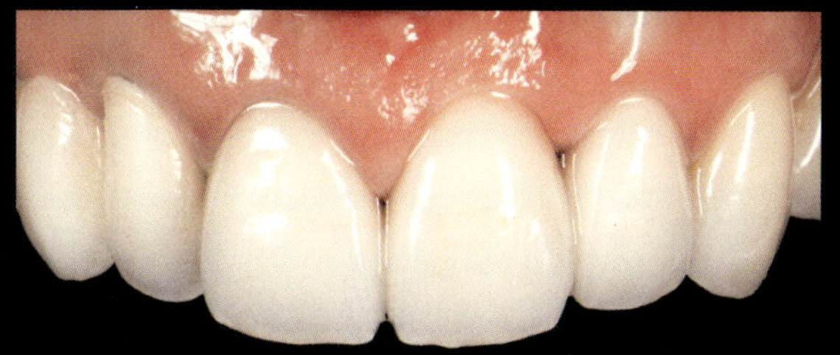

8 years later

Case study 3: Immediate loading of an ovate pontic

If no hard tissue is present in the extraction wound, autogenous bone graft or alloplastic augmentation material is transplanted in order to prevent the loss of alveolar bone. In this case, an ovate pontic was placed immediately after extraction. Since the extraction wound was infected, curettage of the cavity was repeated after one week of antibiotic treatment.

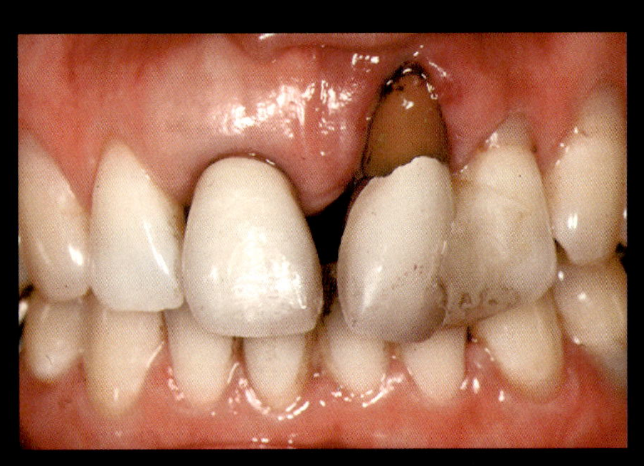

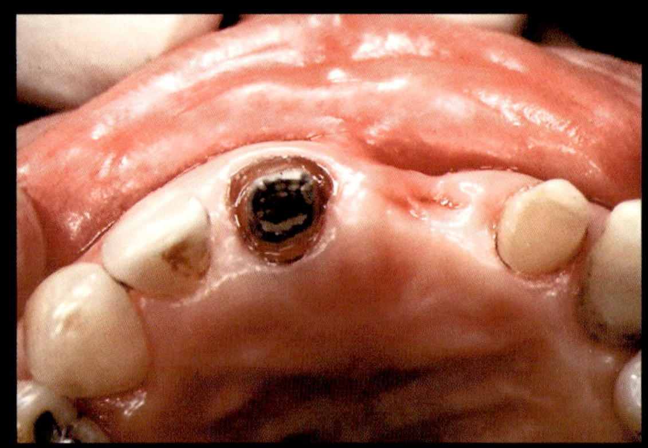

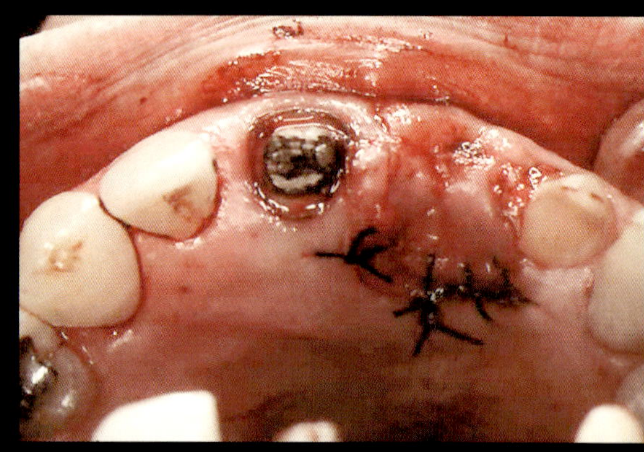

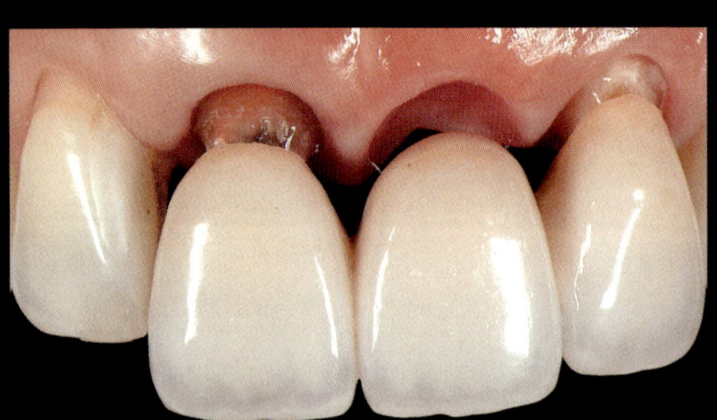

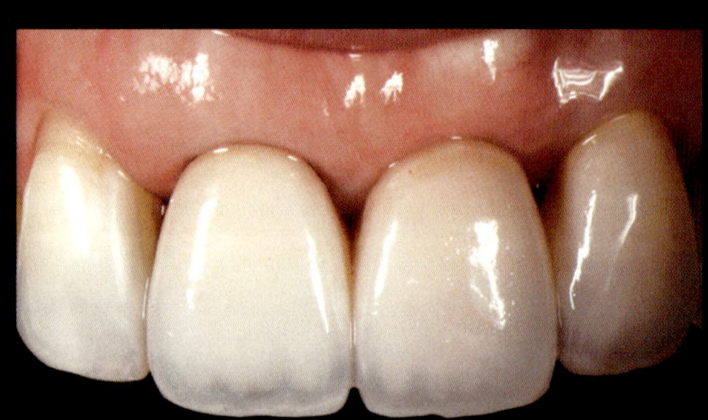

Final restoration

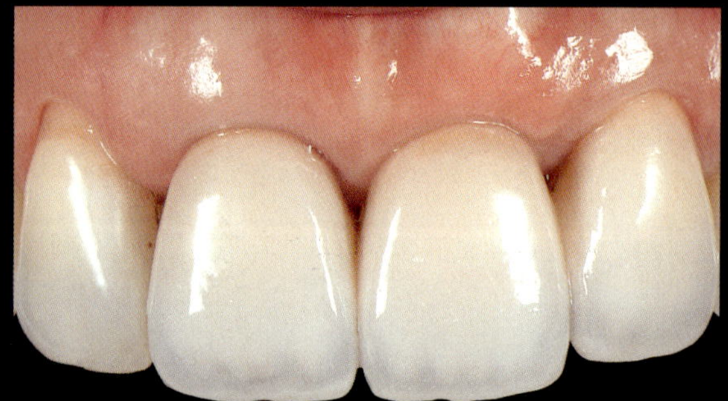

6 years later

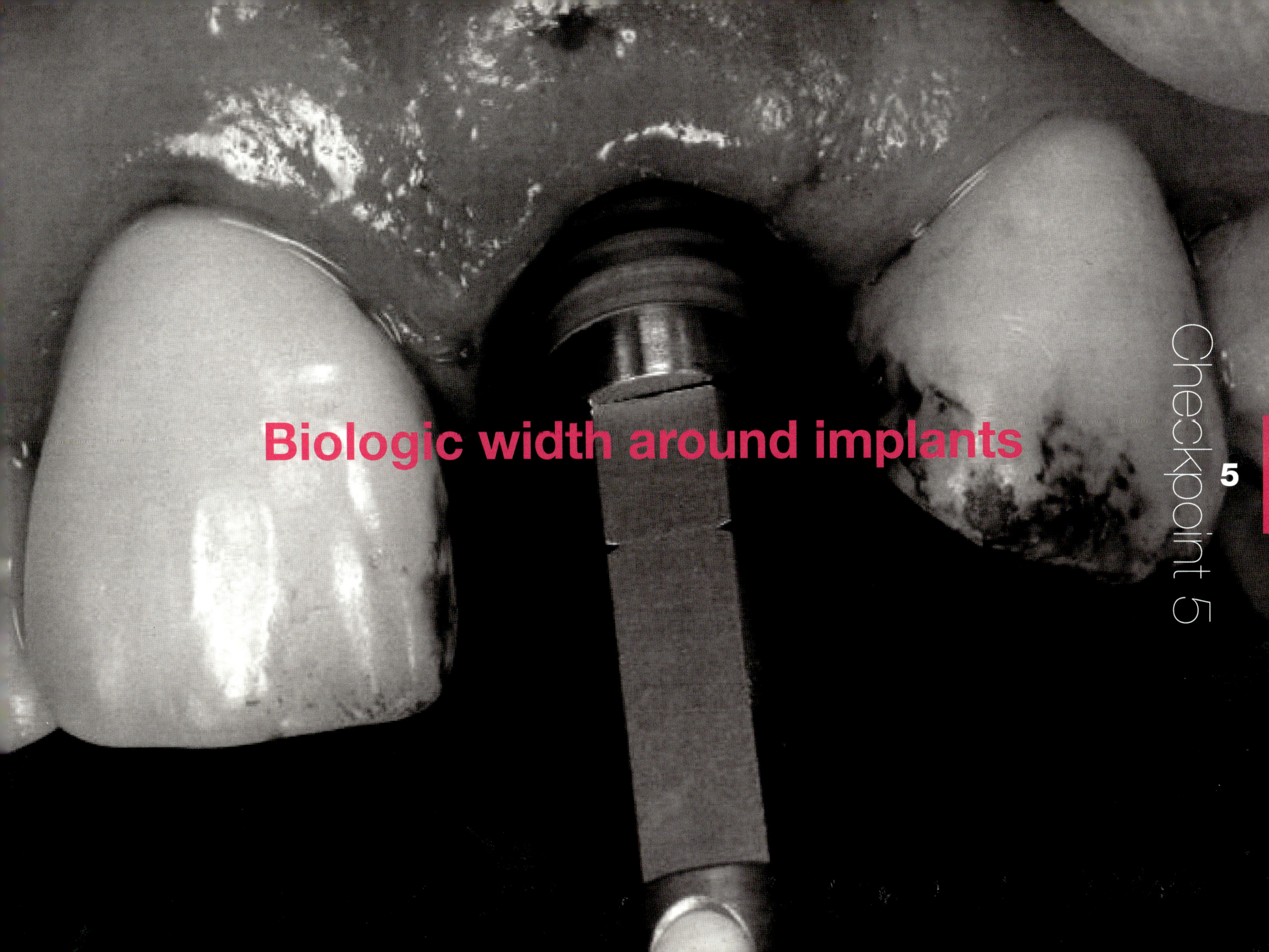

Biologic width around implants

Checkpoint 5

The relationship between implants and the tissues surrounding them (biologic width) was the focus of a number of studies published from the 1990s to the early 2000s. Most of these studies came to the conclusion that the amount of peri-implant tissue absorbed is around 1 mm depending on the surgical technique, the time of surgery, and the type of implant used.
The results are compiled into four main points.

(1) Biologic width around an implant: ca. 4.0 mm (sulcus: 1 mm; junctional epithelium: 1.5 mm; connective tissue attachment: 1.5 mm)
(2) In both delayed and immediate loading, up to 1 mm of hard and soft tissue can be absorbed before the time of crown placement.
(3) Biologic width is not influenced by the type or consistency of the implant surface.
(4) Biologic width is not affected by early or late functional loading of the implant.

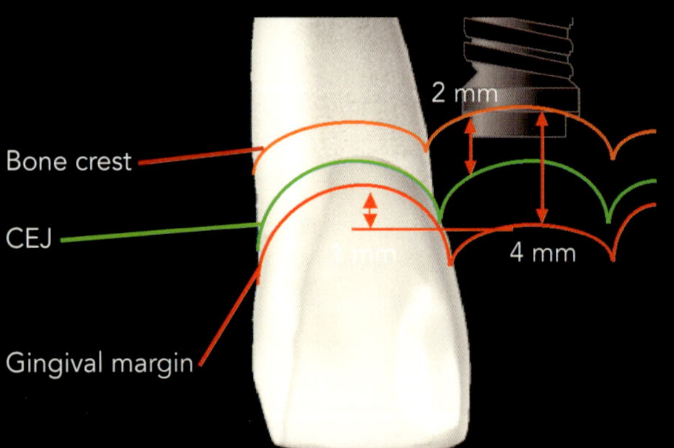

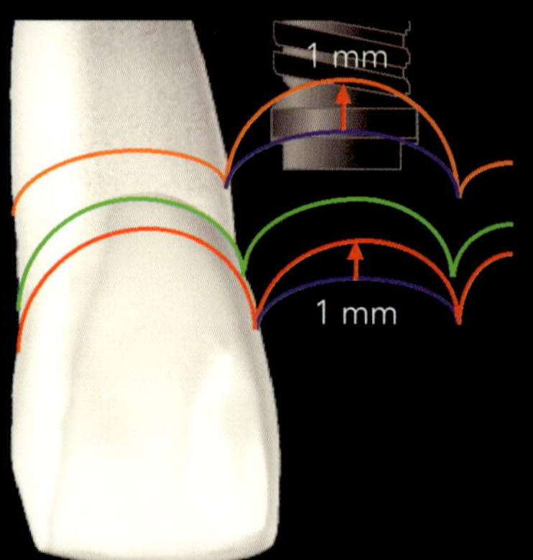

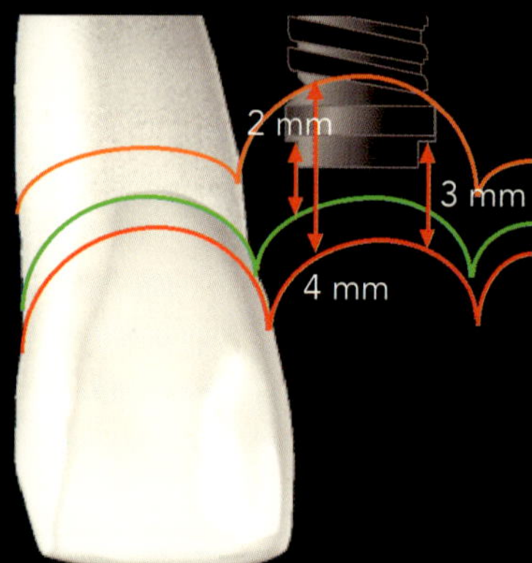

Clinical guidelines

Types in which the margin between the implant and abutment lies at the level of the alveolar crest Insertion depth criteria

Up to 1 mm of hard and soft tissue can be absorbed after an implant has been inserted. Implants should therefore be inserted in such a way that the implant platform lies 2 mm below the cemento-enamel junction (equivalent to the crown margin) and 4 mm below the gingival margin of the restored tooth. This requires the presence of sufficient hard tissue at this level. The gingival margin can also be expected to recede by up to 1 mm. A coronal gingival margin of 1 mm is therefore required.
The gingival margin and the alveolar crest recede by about 1 mm during or after implant loading. The implant platform and the osseous crest will ultimately lie 3 mm and 4 mm below the gingival margin. This corresponds to a biologic width of 4 mm.

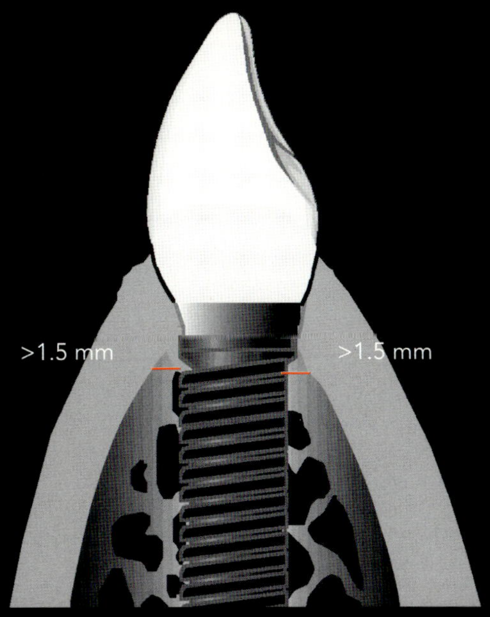

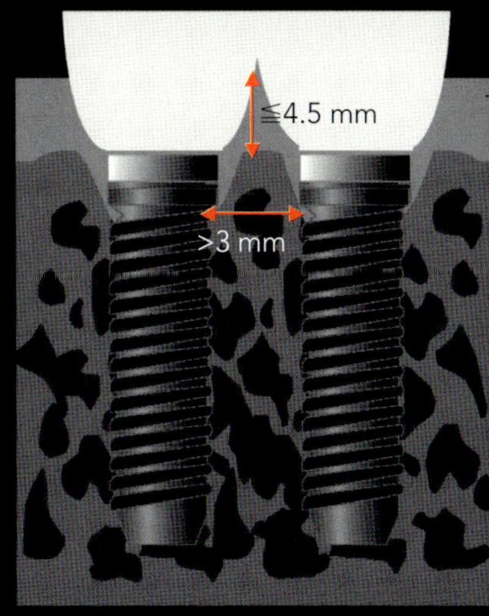

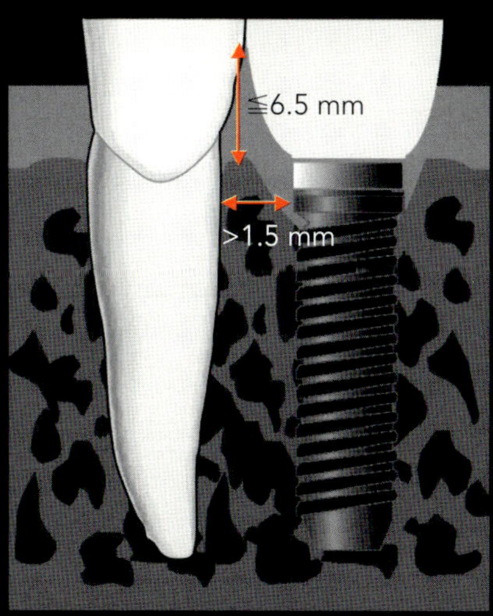

Insertion criteria for the buccolingual dimension

The recipient site is adequate if more than 1.5 mm of bone is present in the buccal (labial) and lingual (palatal) dimension.

Insertion criteria for the mesiodistal dimension

The distance between an implant and natural teeth must be greater than 1.4 mm, and the distance between two adjacent implants must be greater than 3 mm.

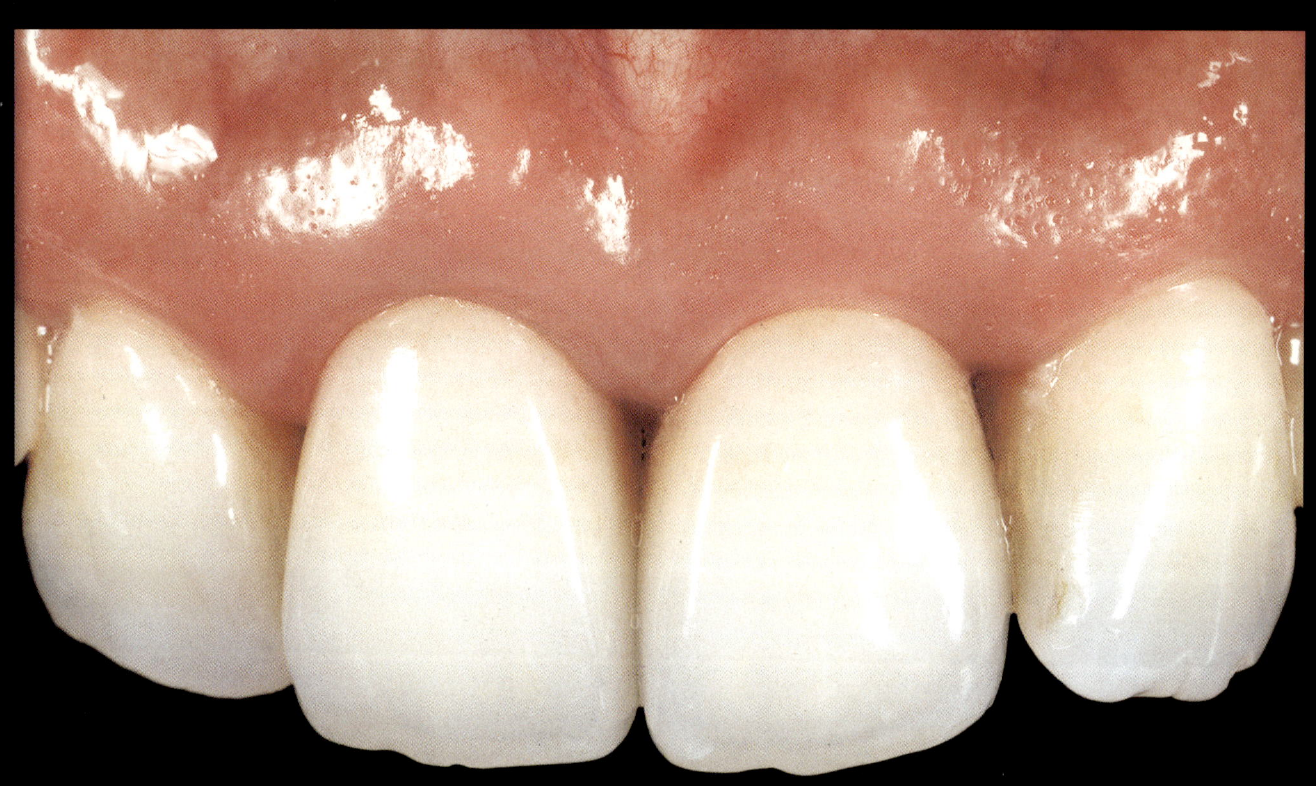

5 years later

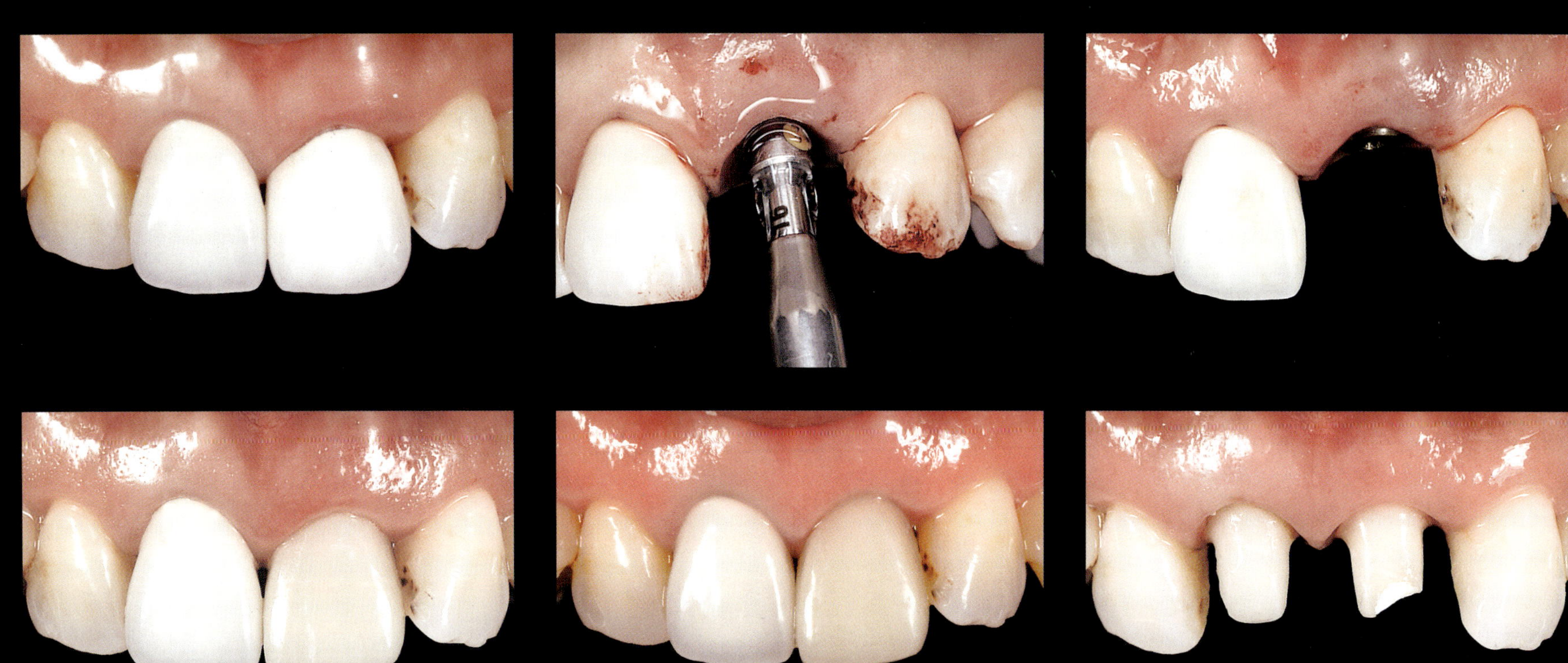

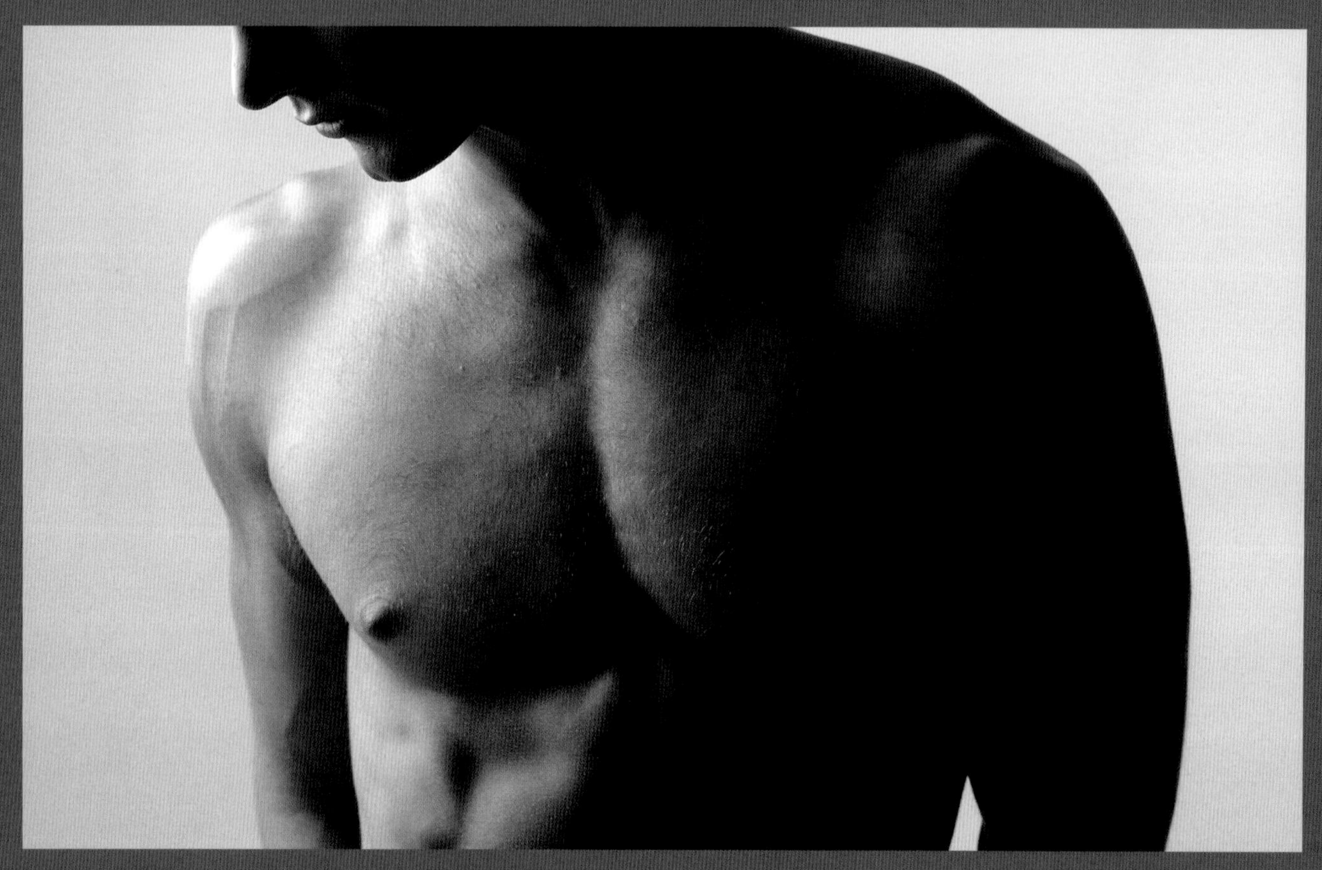

6 Esthetic integration

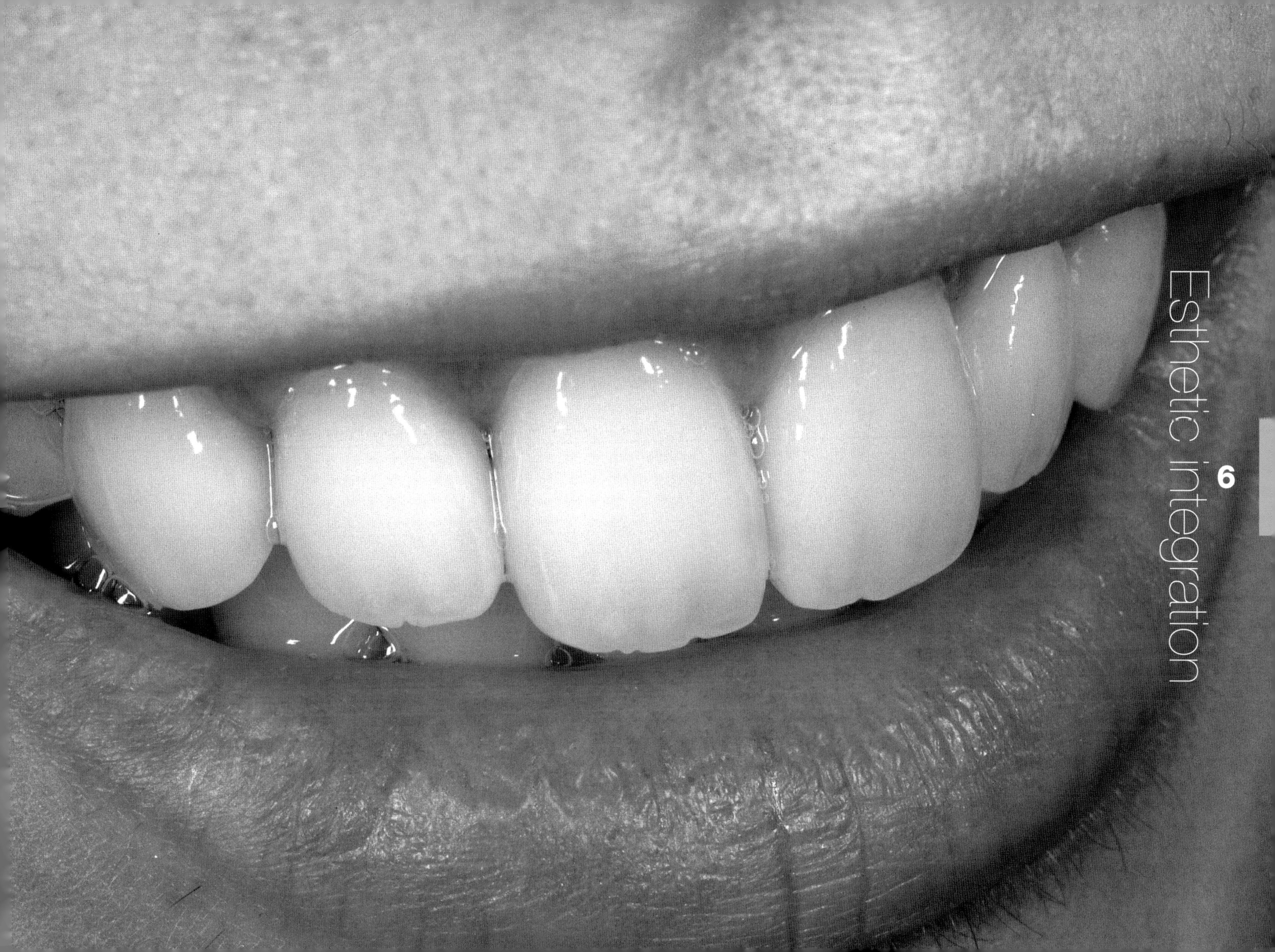

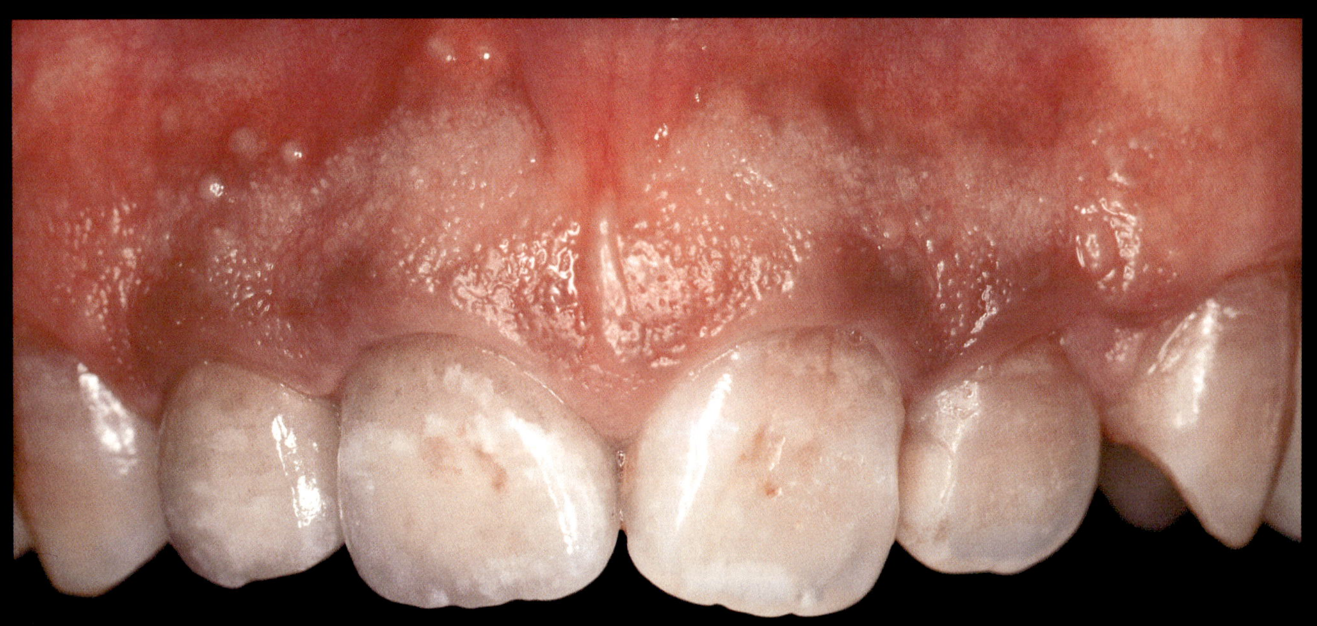

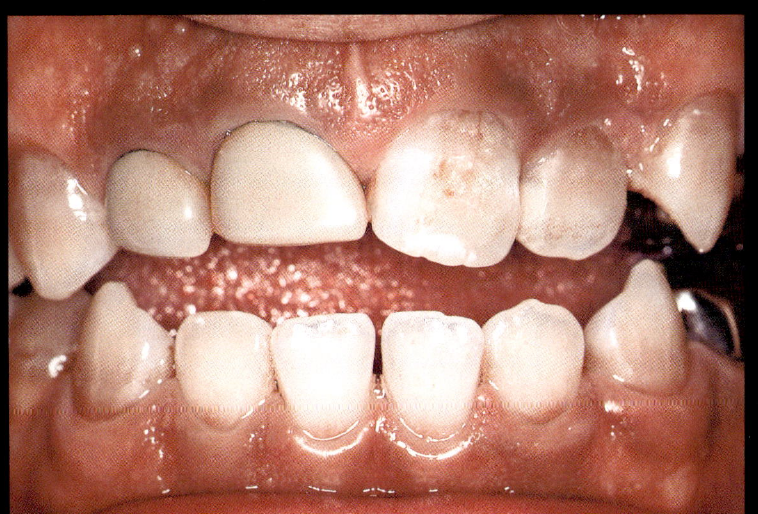

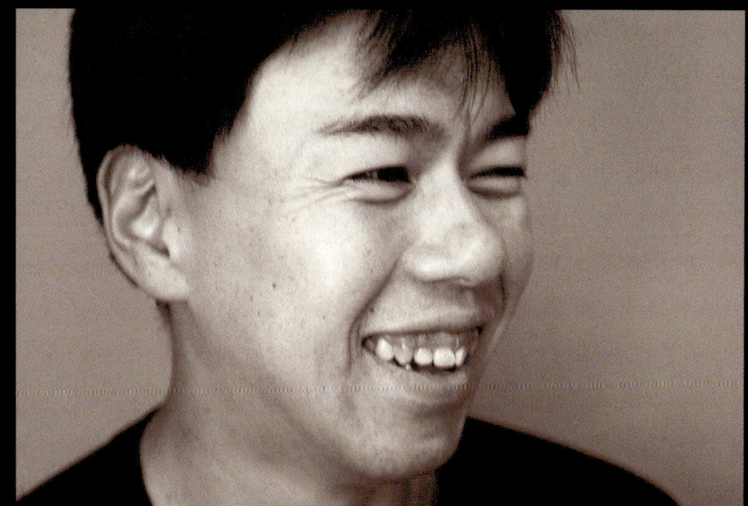

Subjective esthetic integration

Beauty is a perceptual phenomenon that is subject to change over time and varies from one culture to another. This patient wanted his right central and lateral incisors to look like they had in the past.

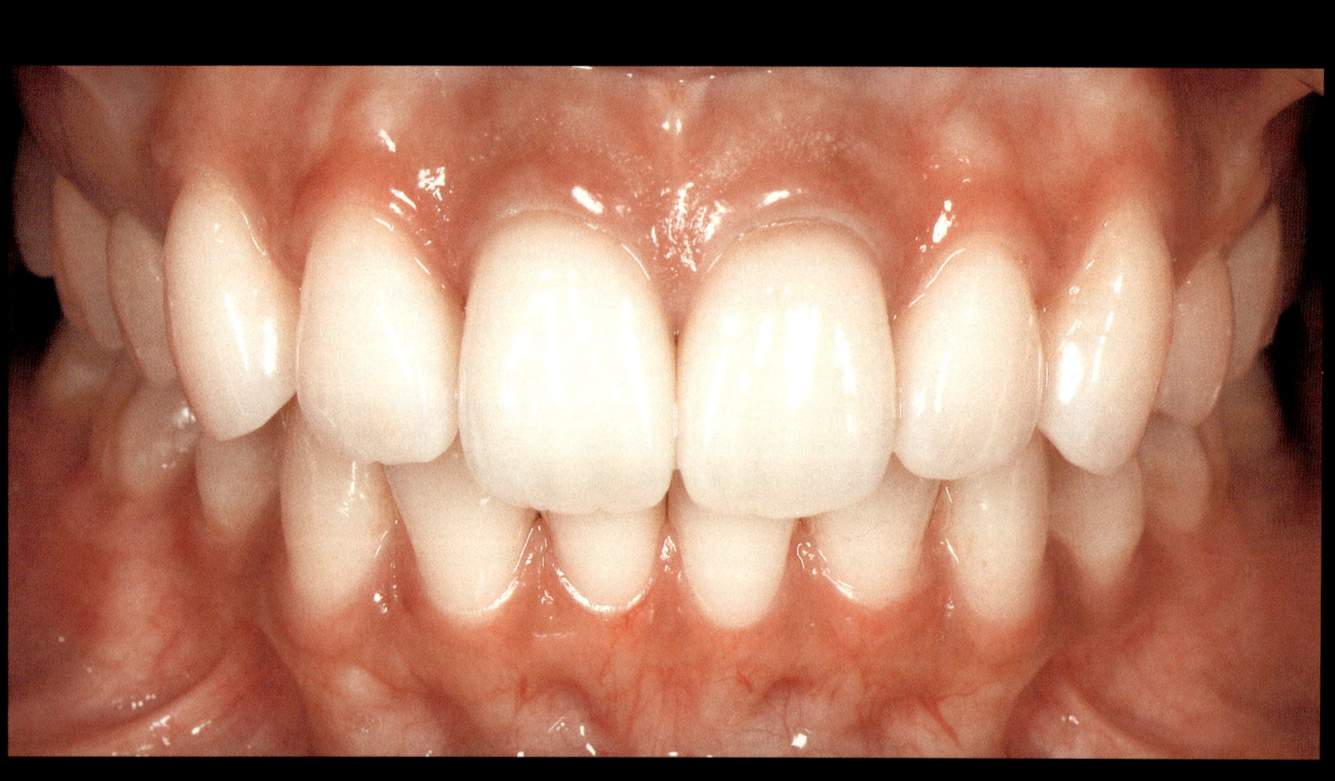

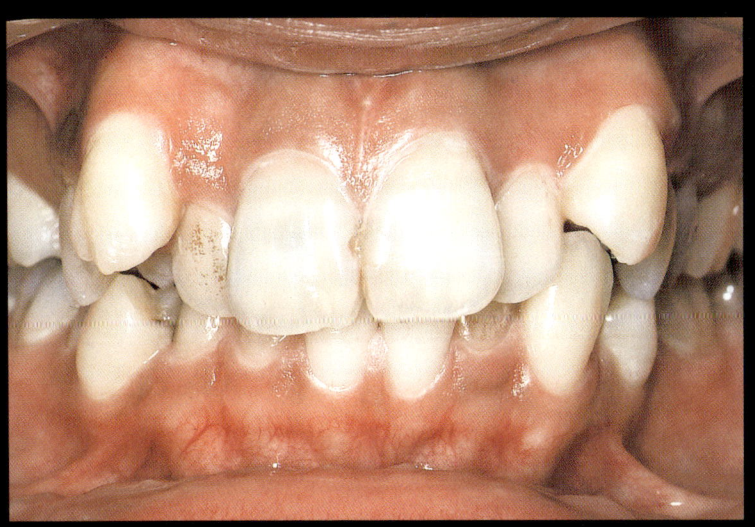

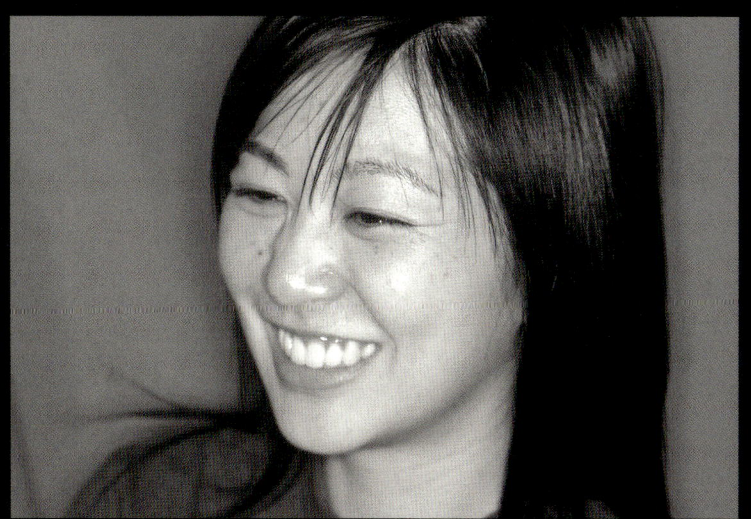

Objective esthetic integration

Although nature does not produce symmetry in geometric perfection, general rules based on objective morphometry can enhance the charm of beauty.

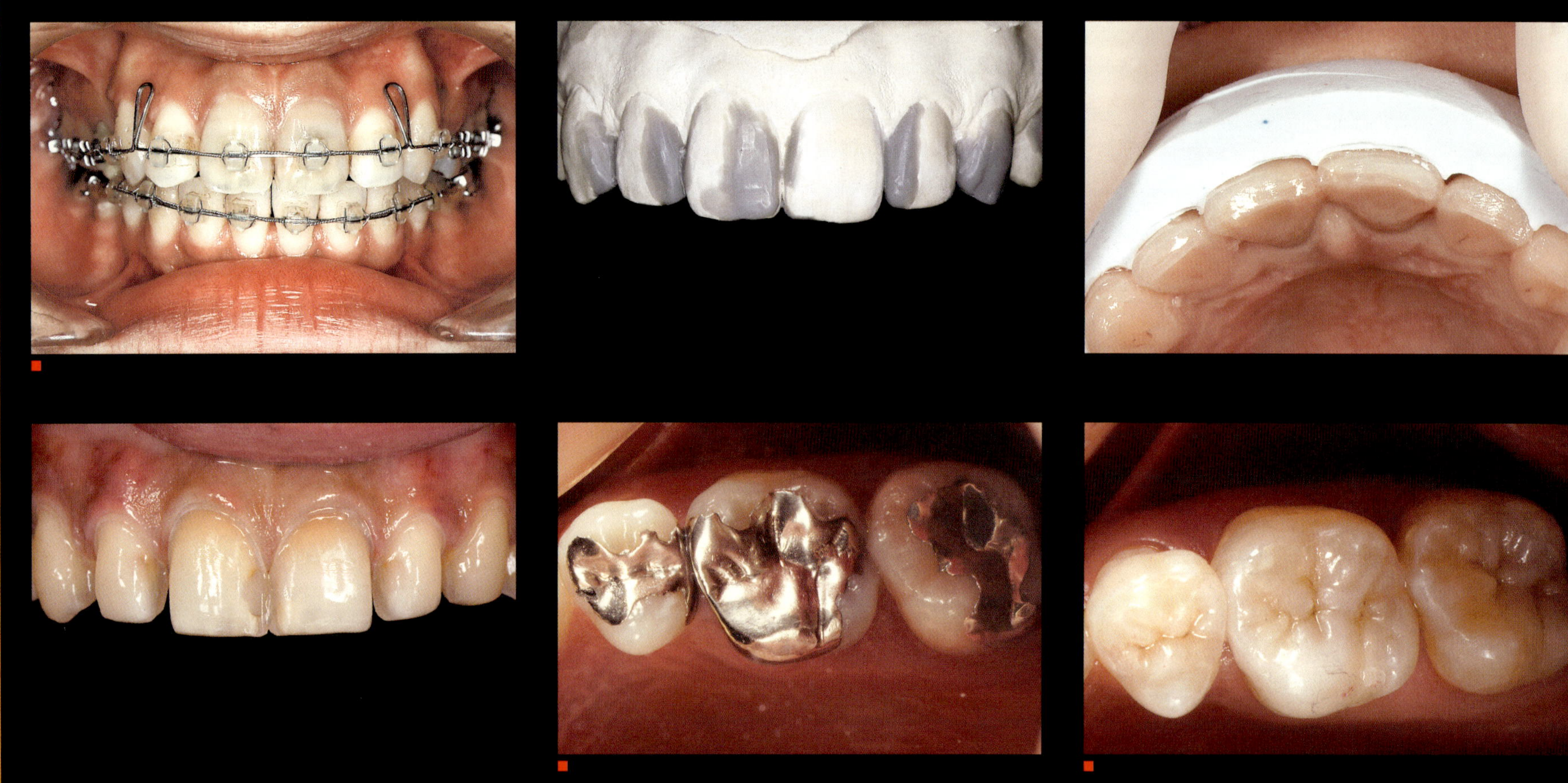

After this patient had completed orthodontic treatment, ceramic veneers, inlays and onlays were used to restore the anterior teeth in order to achieve harmonization of the width and color of the teeth.

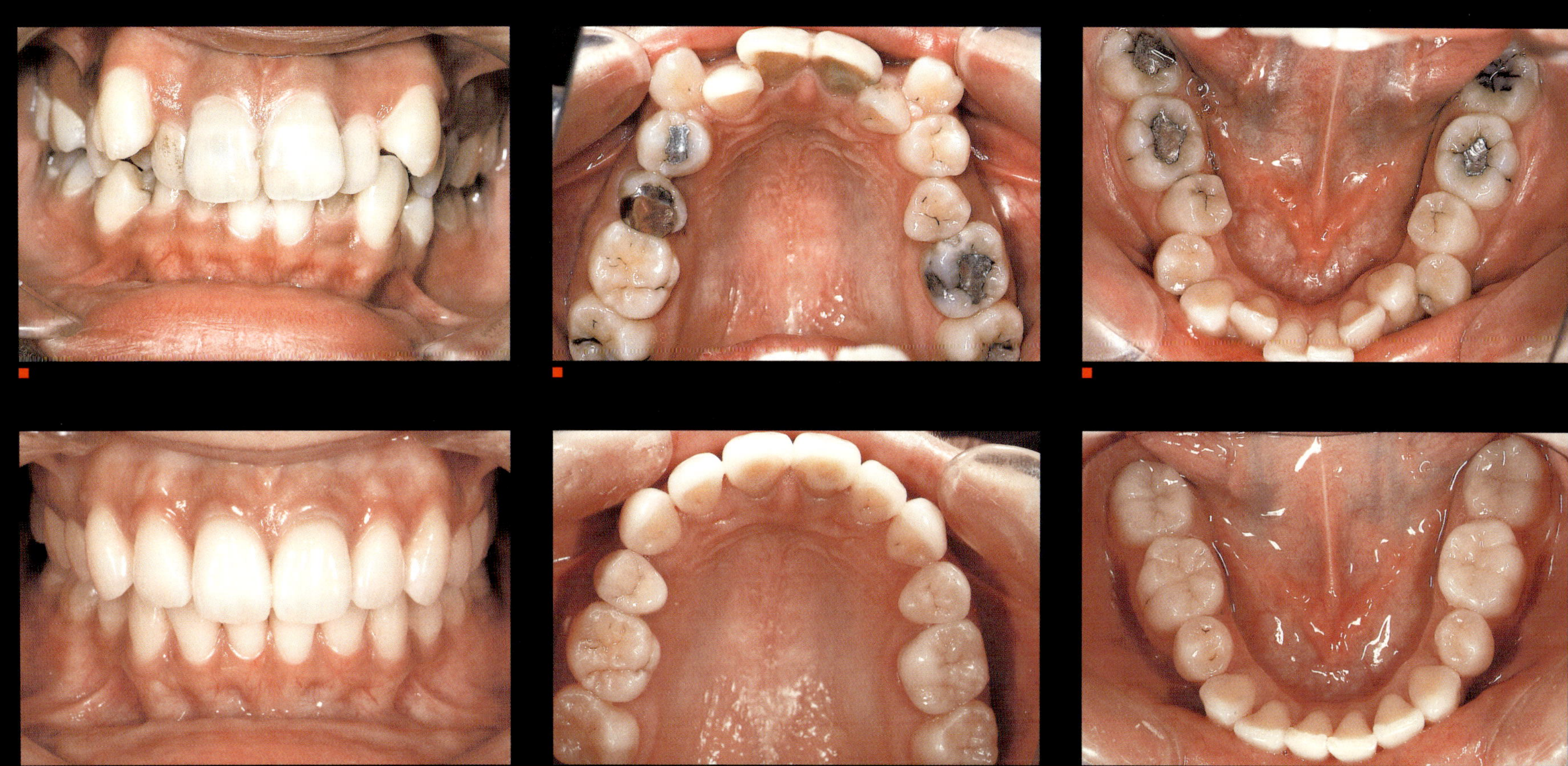

Ceramic veneers, inlays and onlays

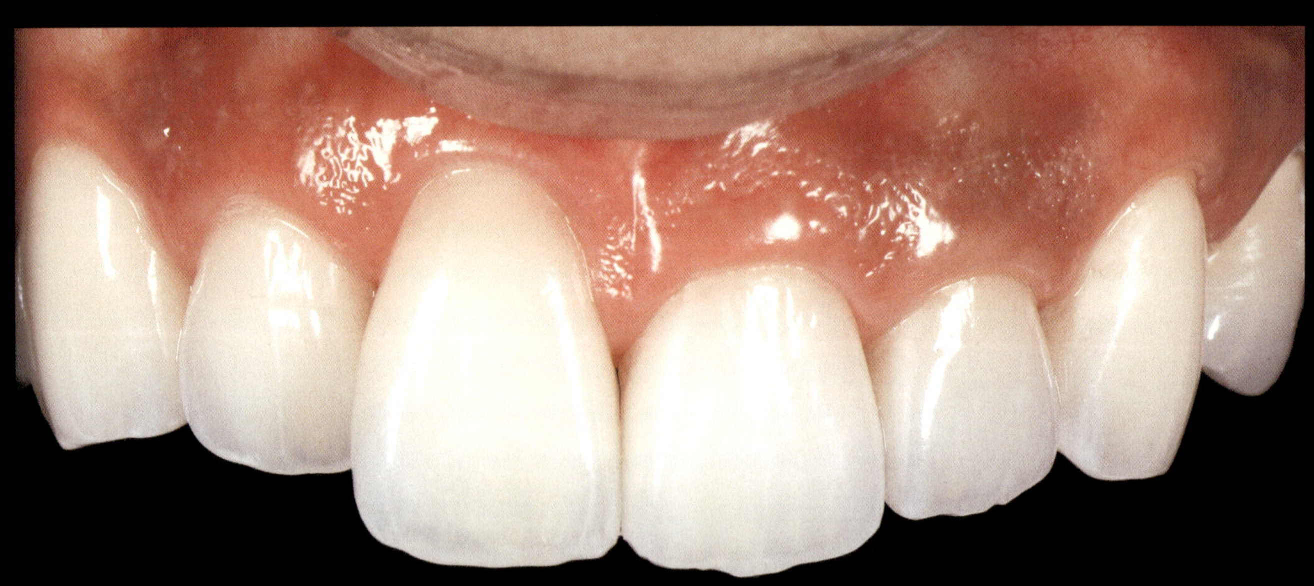

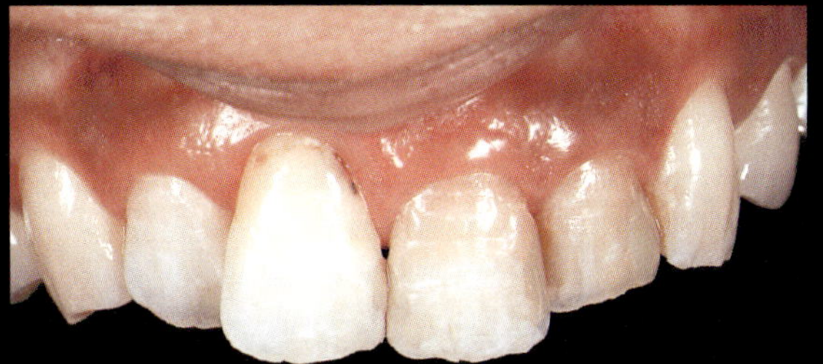

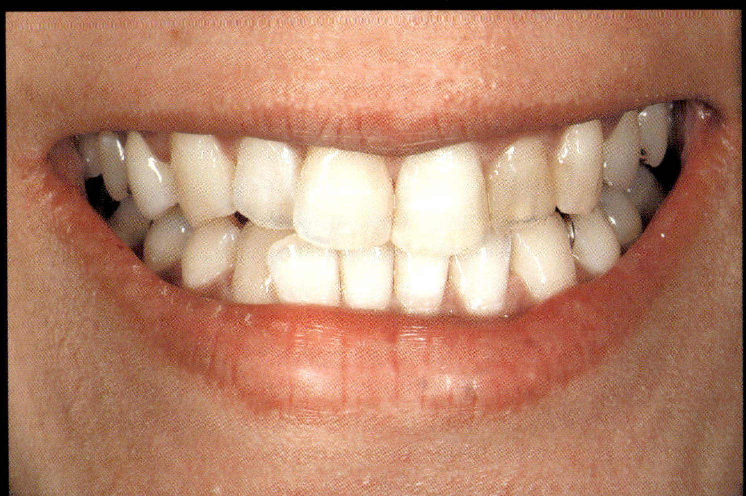

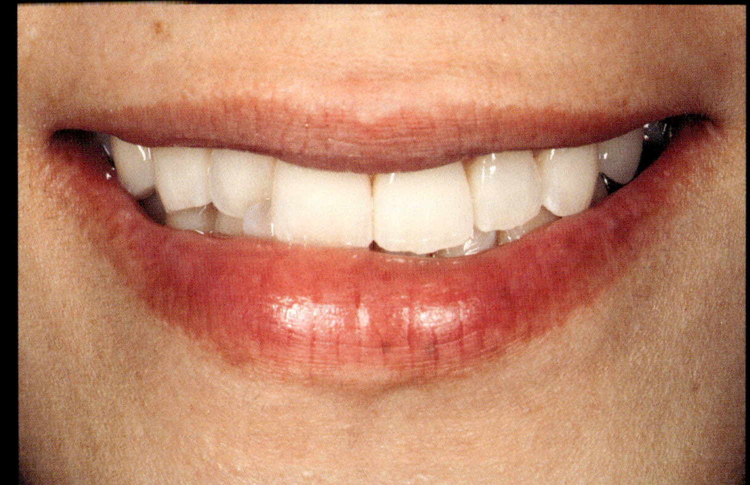

Esthetic integration with limitations to treatment

Some patients do not consent to all measures regarded by the restorative dentist as necessary for achievement of the desired esthetic outcome. Since this patient wanted fast results, ceramic veneers were used to improve tooth color, width and axial direction in an attempt to meet the patient's expectations. She was pleased with the results.

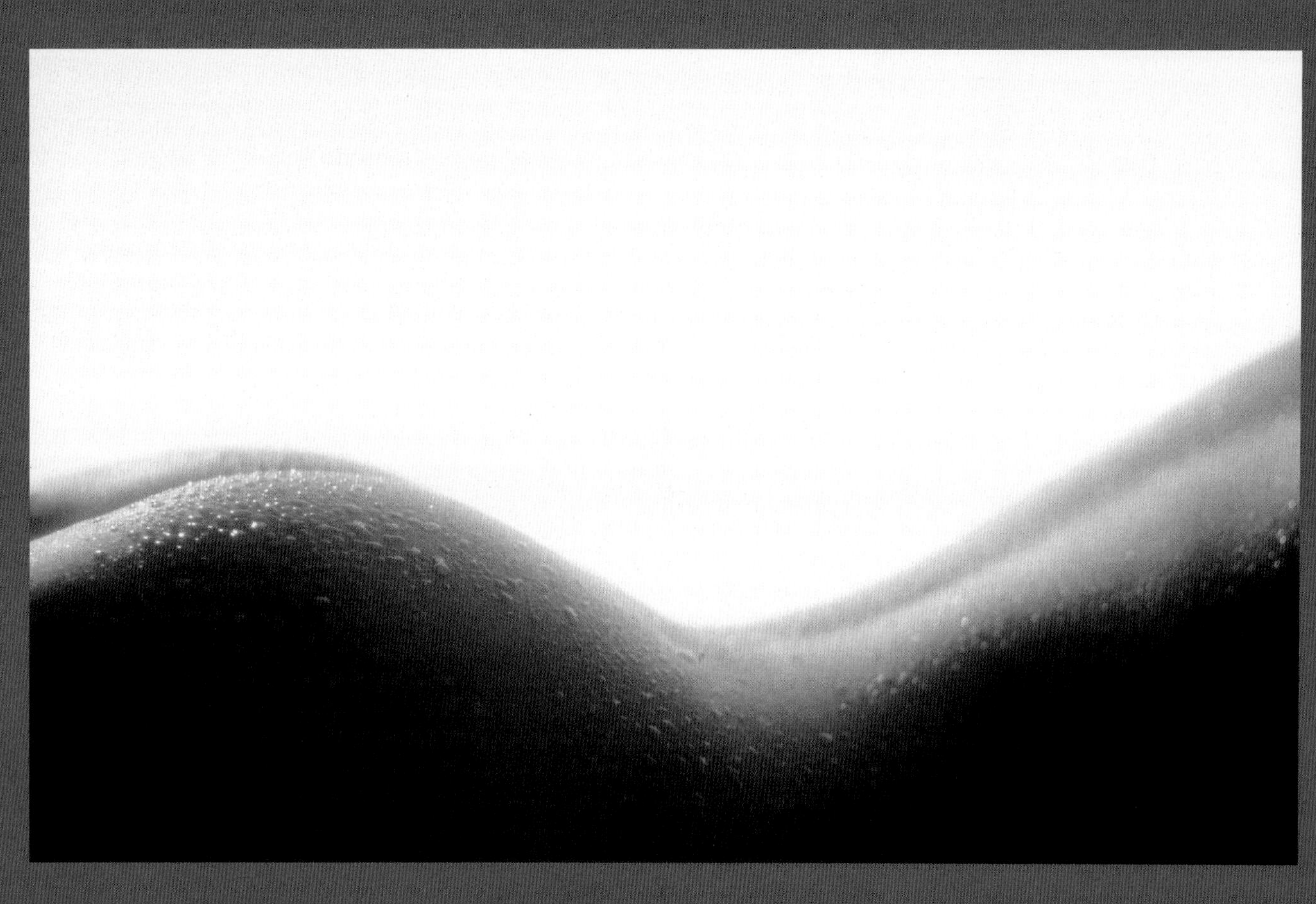

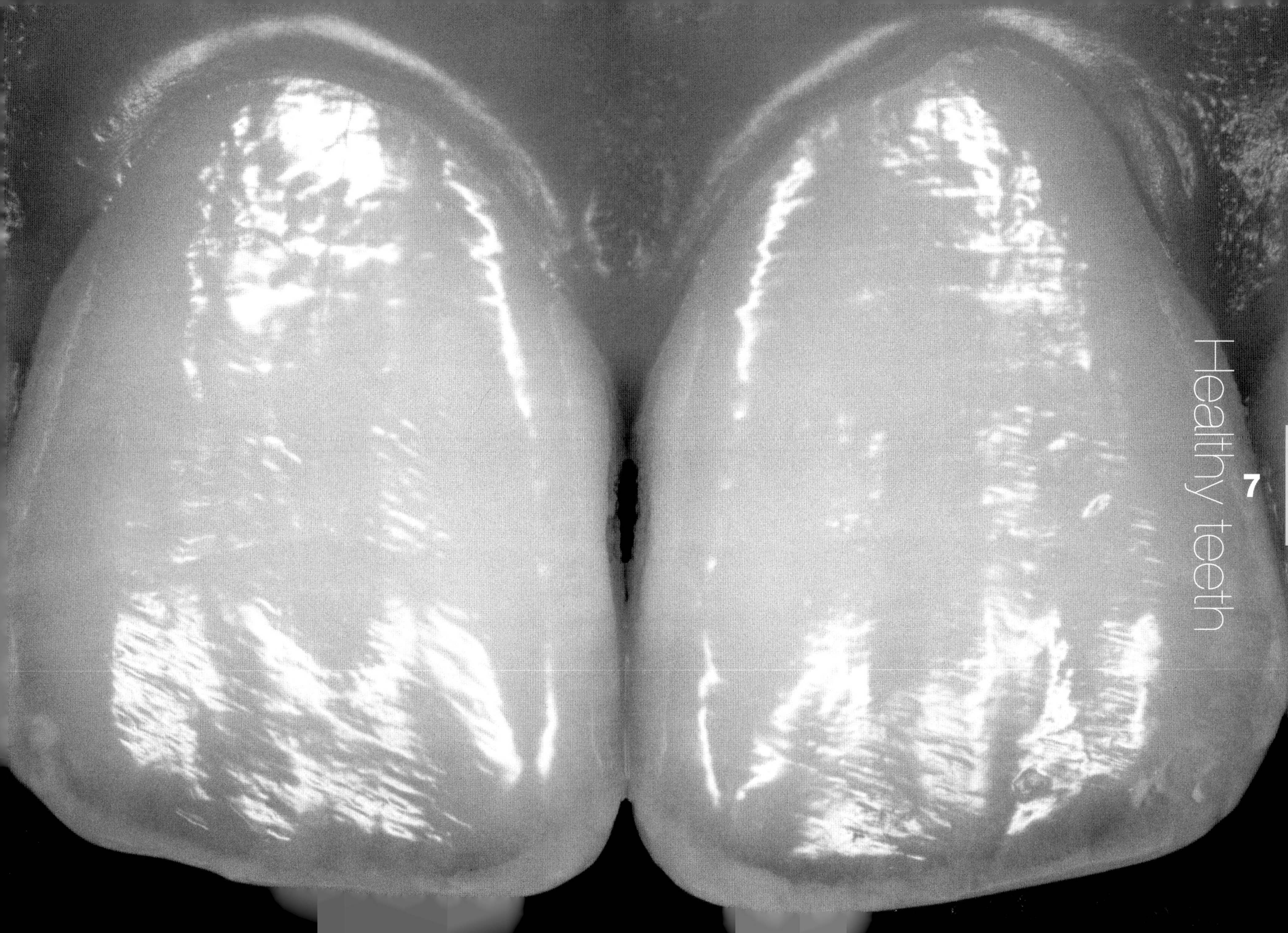

Healthy teeth

Healthy teeth vary in appearance, color, shape, surface structure and other characteristics.

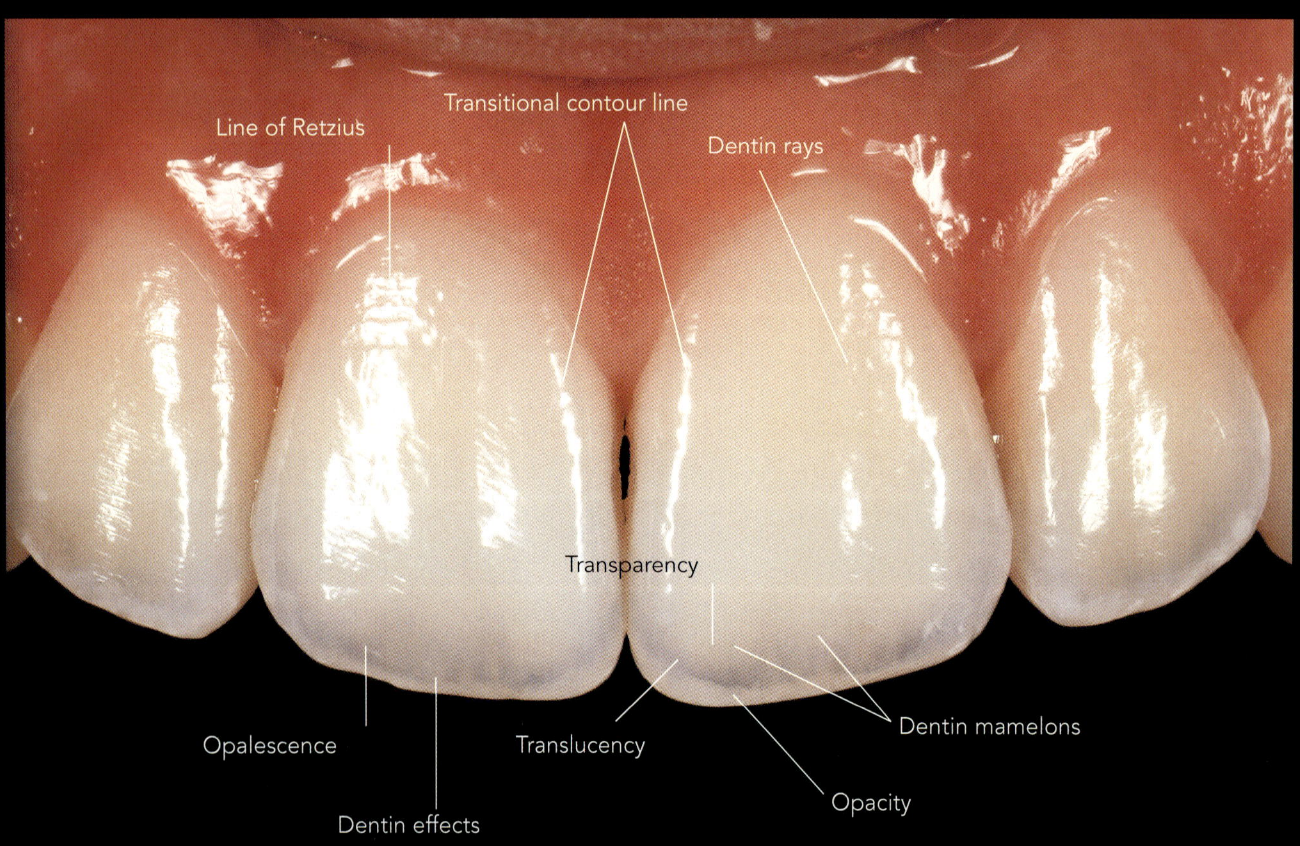

19-year-old female

Color

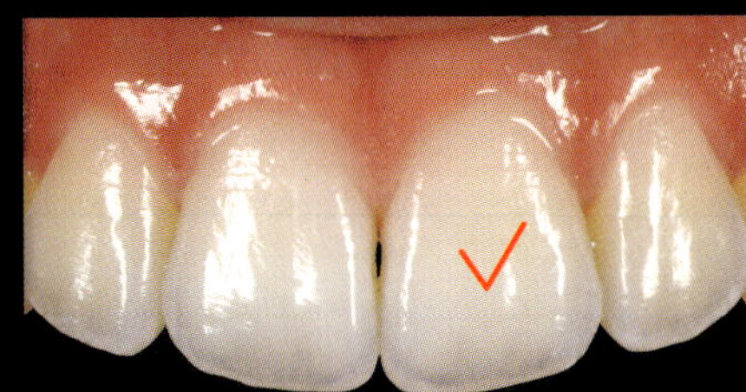

-10% +10%

Value

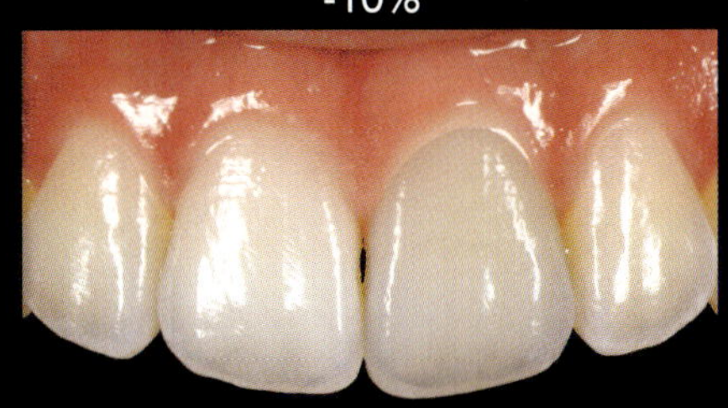

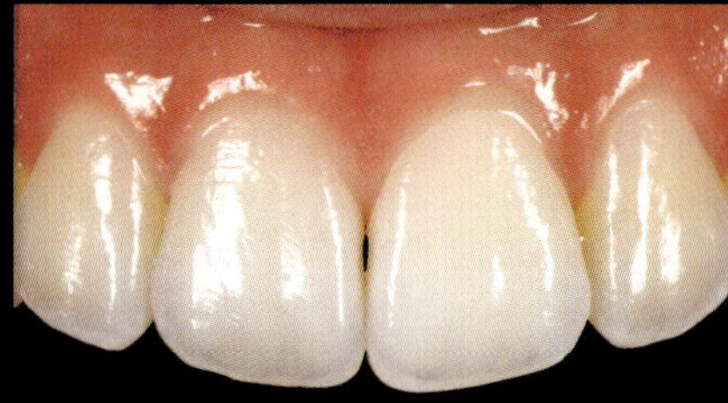

Color

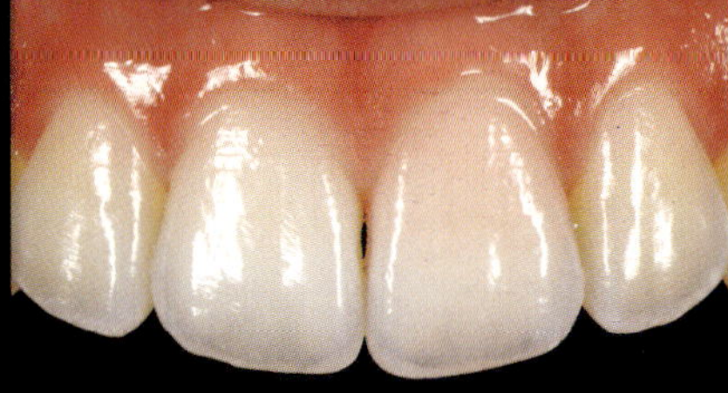

Chroma

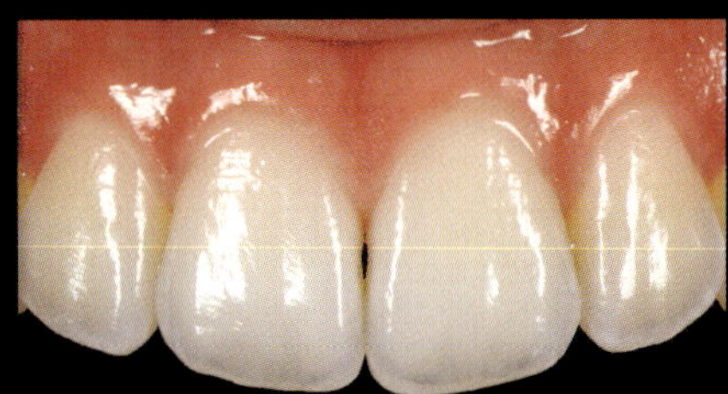

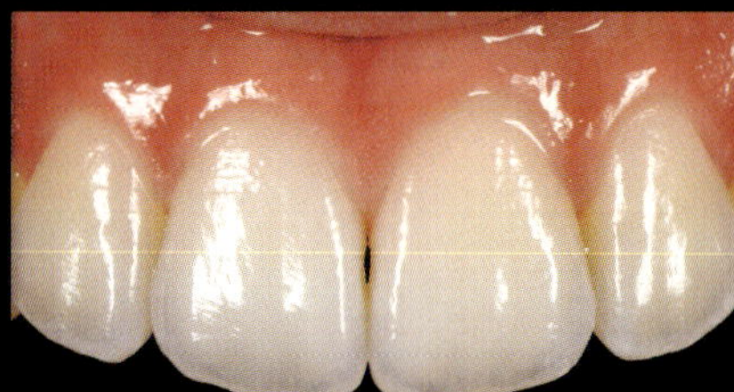

Color

Color perception is determined by three basic characteristics. The color that the human eye sees is most strongly determined by value, less strongly by hue (the color itself), and least by chroma. Each of these variables was changed by ± 10 percent in the left central incisors shown in these photographs.

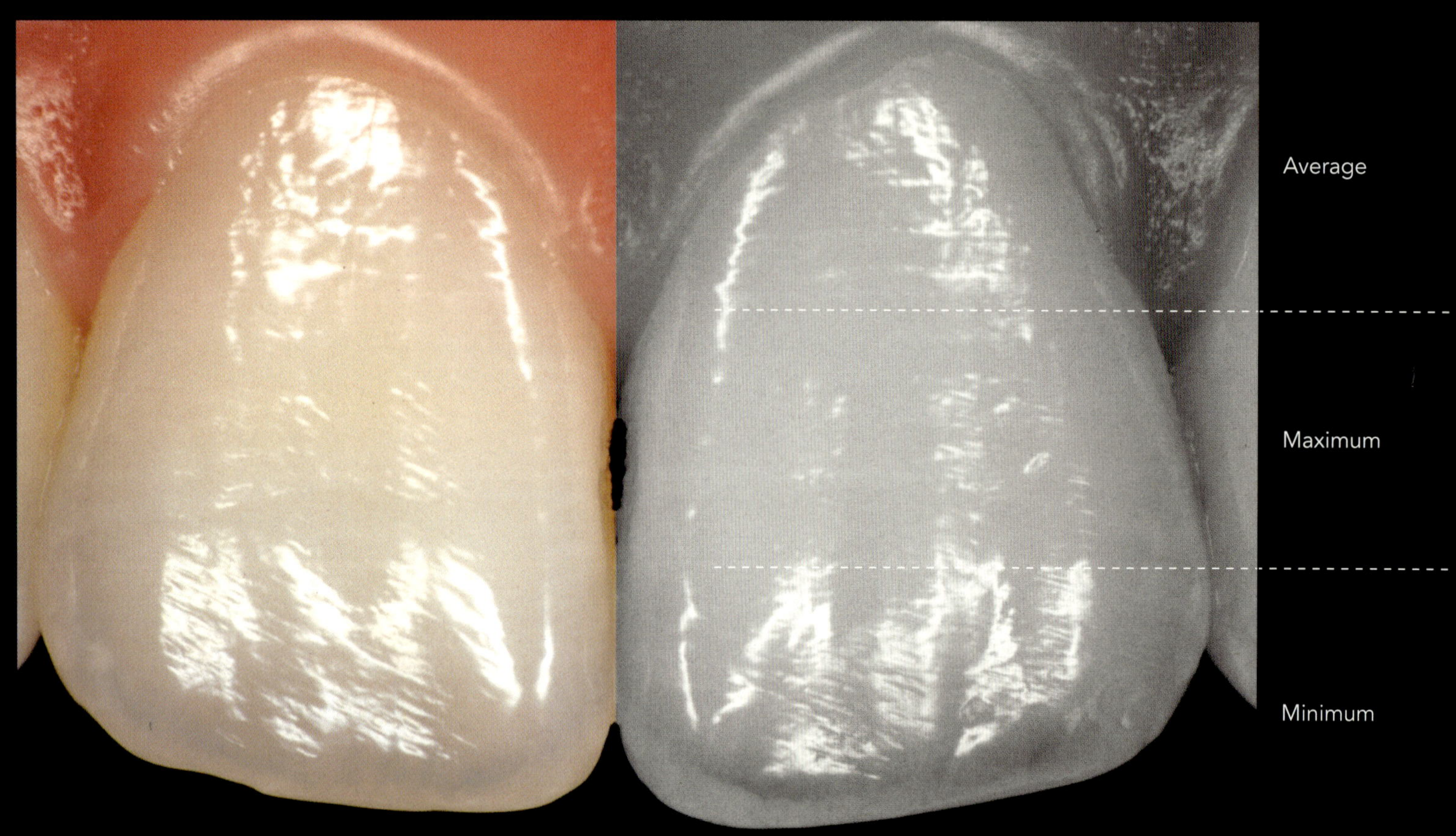

Brightness

The central third of the labial aspect is brightest, and the incisal third is darkest. The cervical third is darker than the central third but lighter than the incisal third.

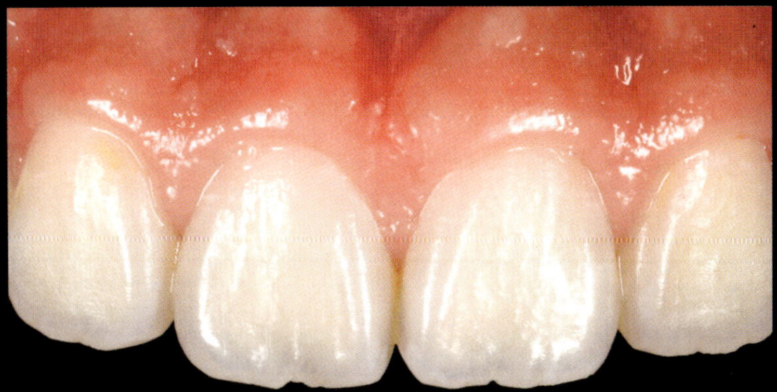

18-year-old female

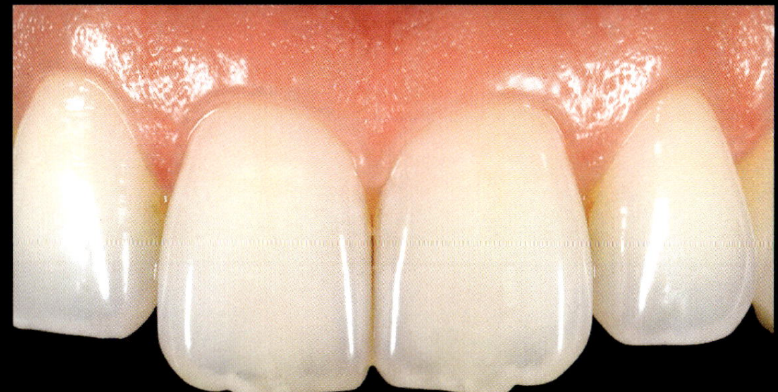

17-year-old female

Surface texture and surface characteristics

It is generally assumed that the tooth surface texture is complex and varied in juveniles and becomes smoother with age. Due to individual differences, however, the surface texture of the teeth varies greatly from one person to another.

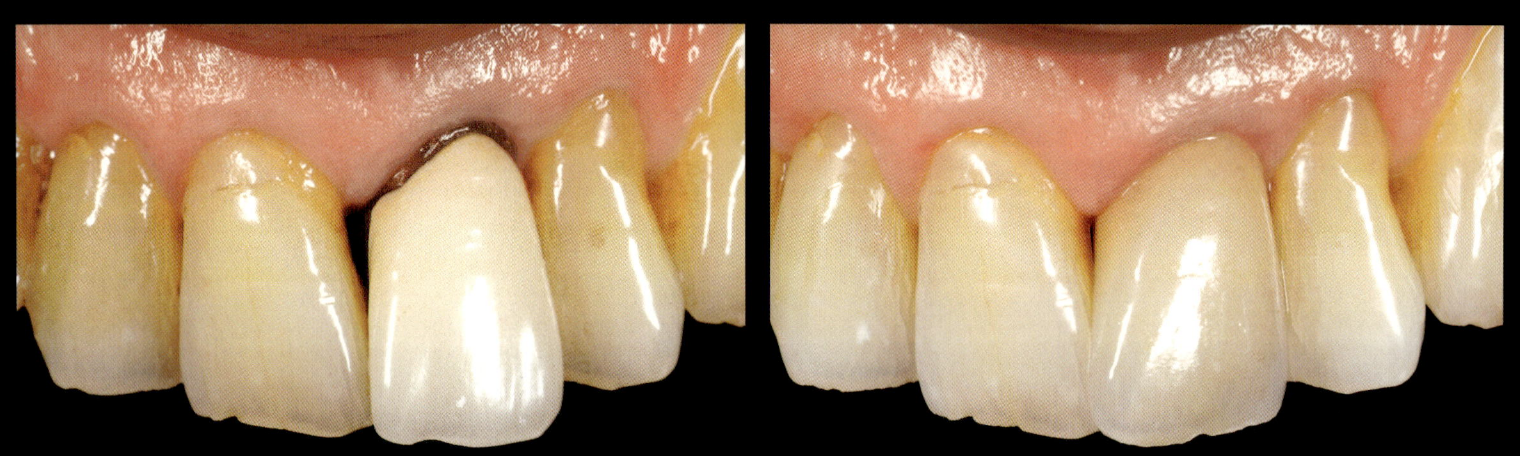

Character

Dental esthetics is a science that attempts to create unobtrusive products.

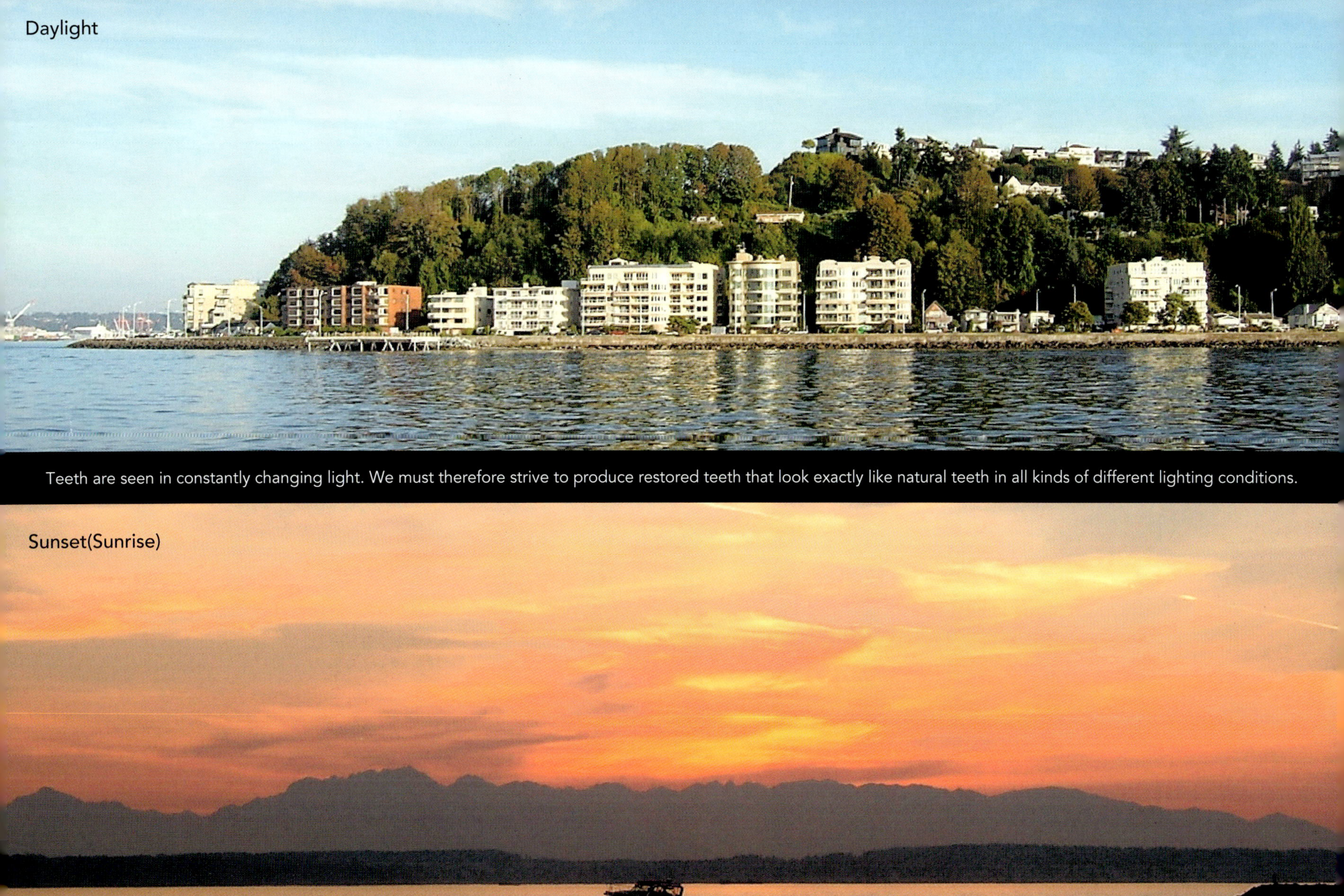

Teeth are seen in constantly changing light. We must therefore strive to produce restored teeth that look exactly like natural teeth in all kinds of different lighting conditions.

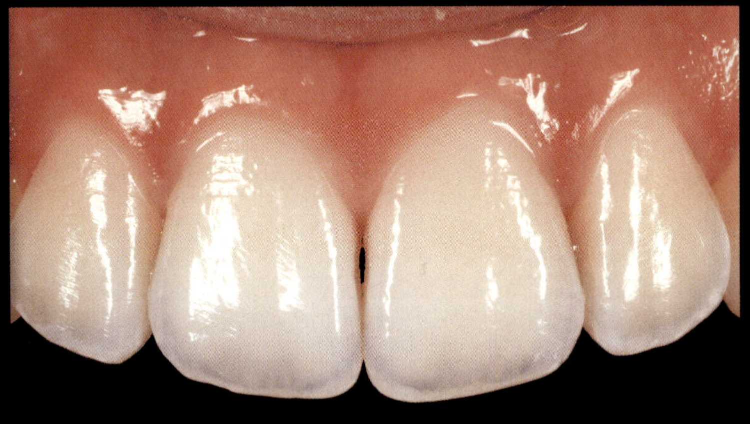

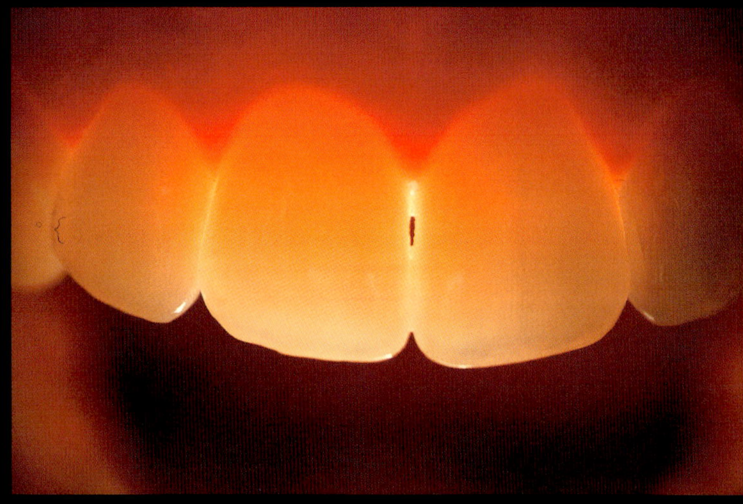

Transparency

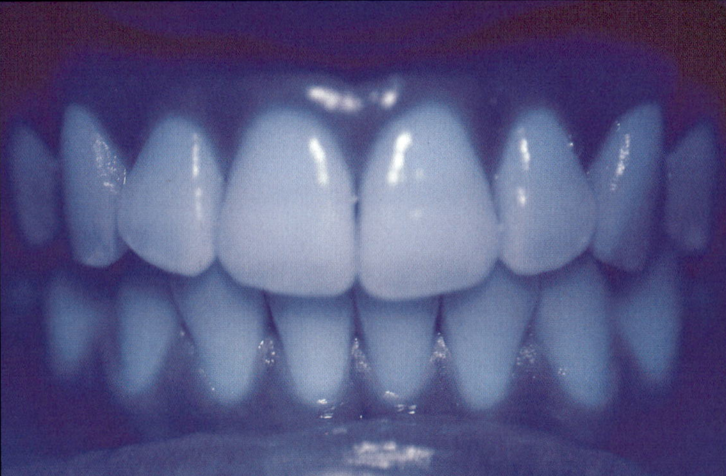

Fluorescence

Intact teeth

Intact teeth as they appear in different lighting conditions (frontlighting, backlighting and infrared light). The brightness of the cervical zone in backlighting is a marked effect. Because of fluorescence, the teeth look strikingly whitish in infrared light.

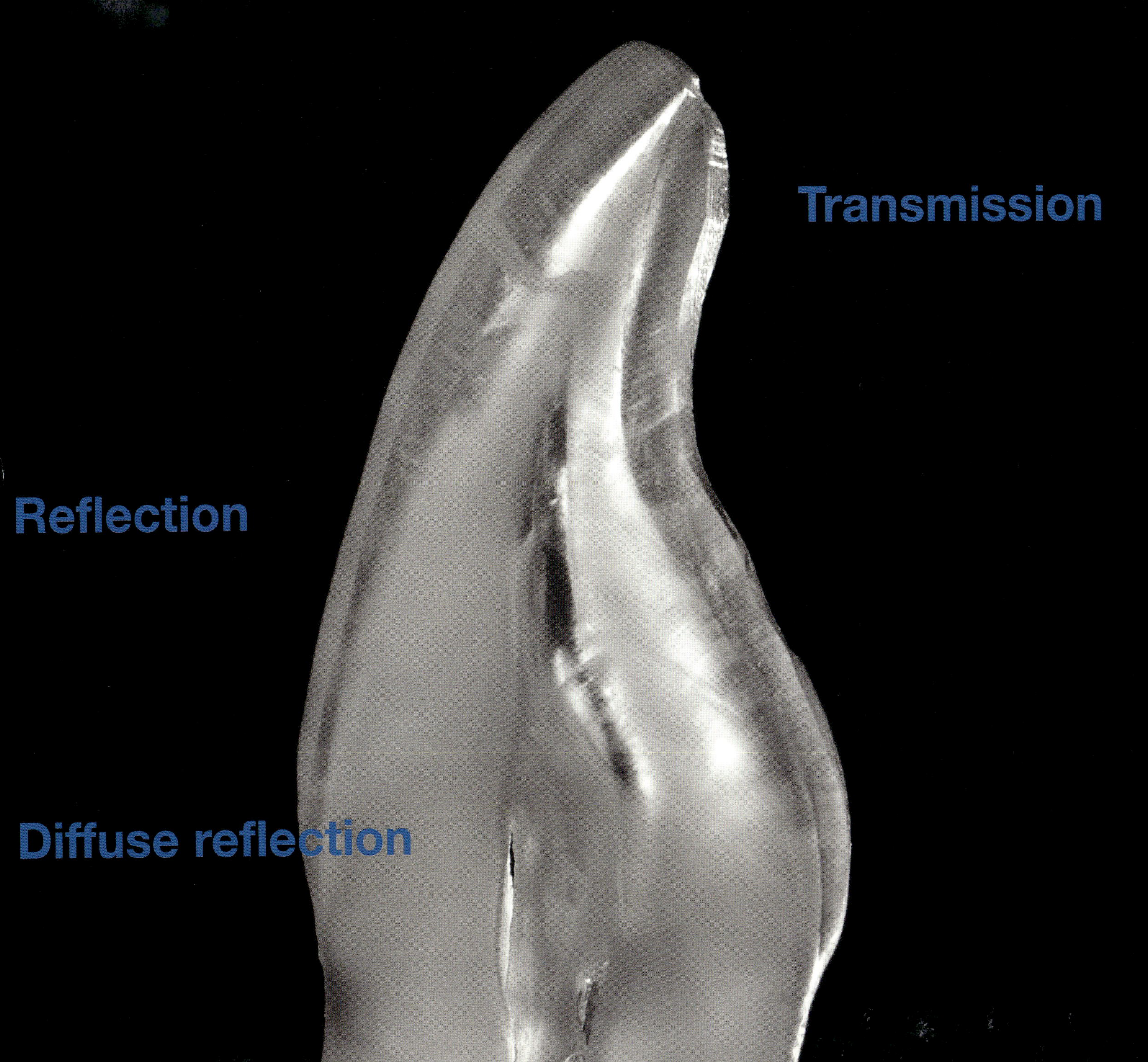
Transmission
Reflection
Diffuse reflection

Healthy natural teeth are perceived as teeth in transillumination as well as in reflected and diffuse light.

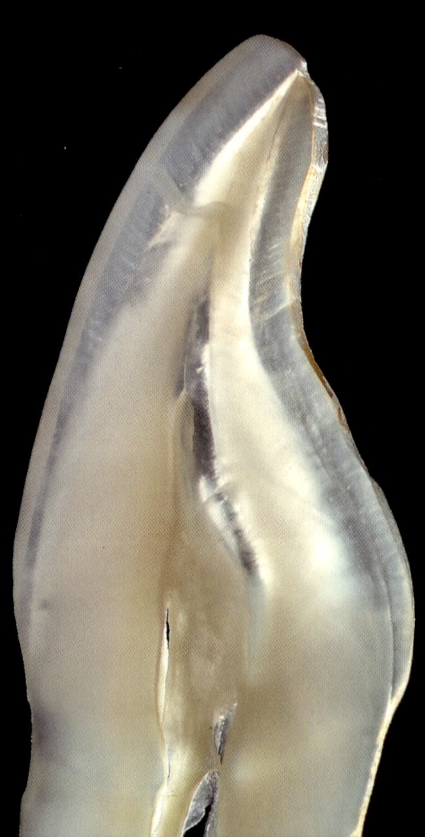

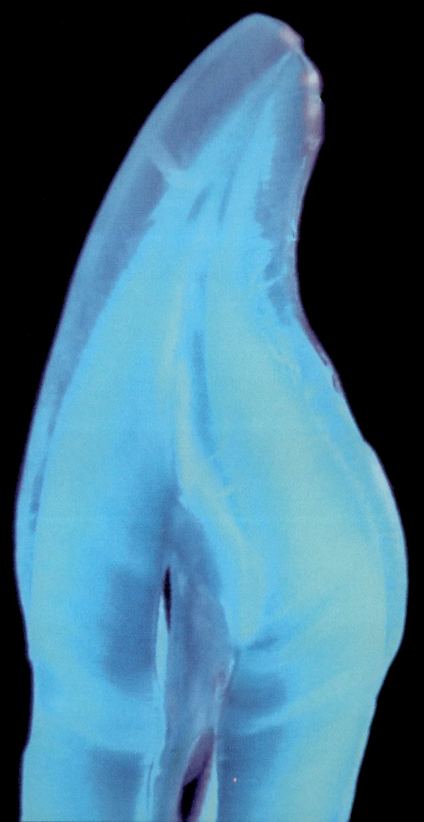

Natural tooth

Thin sections of a maxillary central incisor and a maxillary first molar (page 57) seen in transillumination and in infrared light.

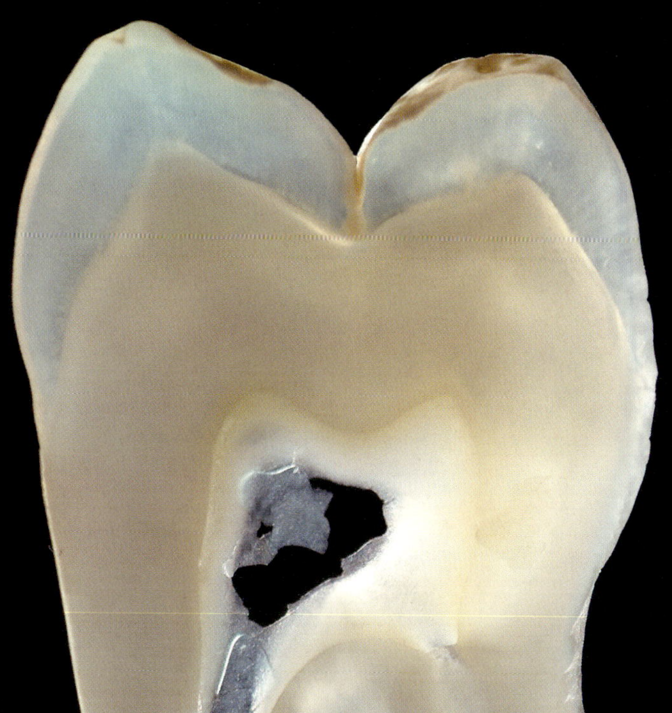

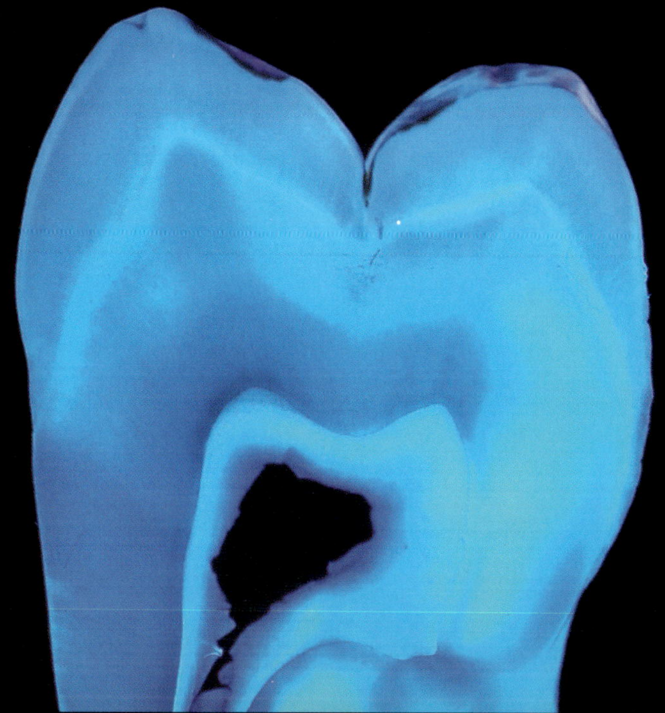

Natural tooth

Fluorescence is strongest at the cemento-dentin junction. Consequently, the caps of all-ceramic crowns and the cement used to attach them must also fluoresce.

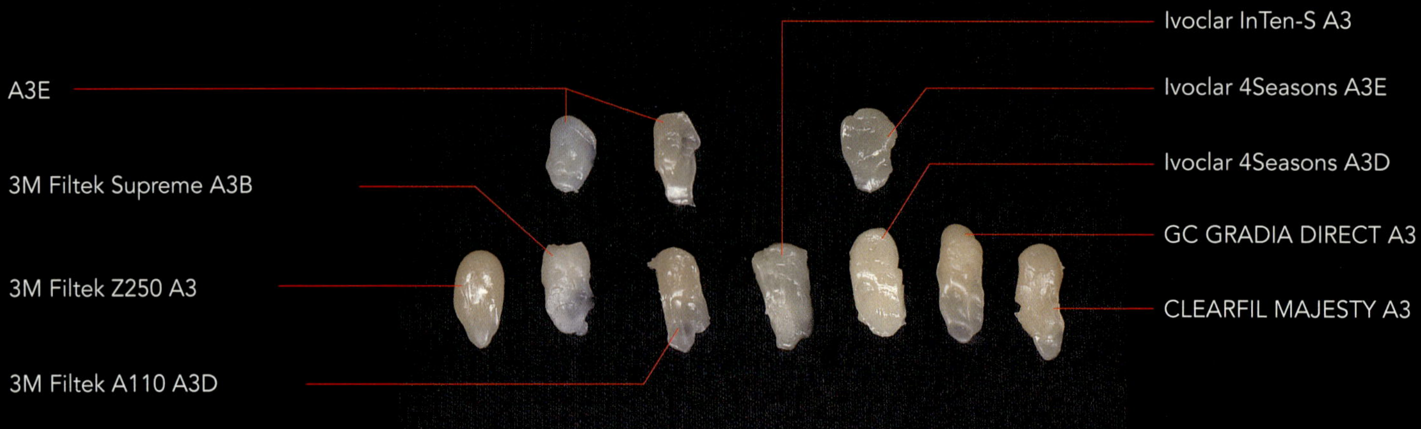

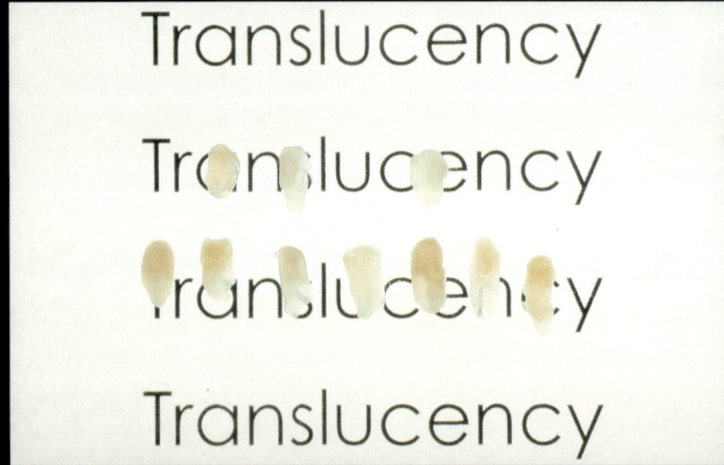

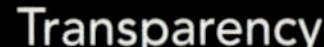
Transparency

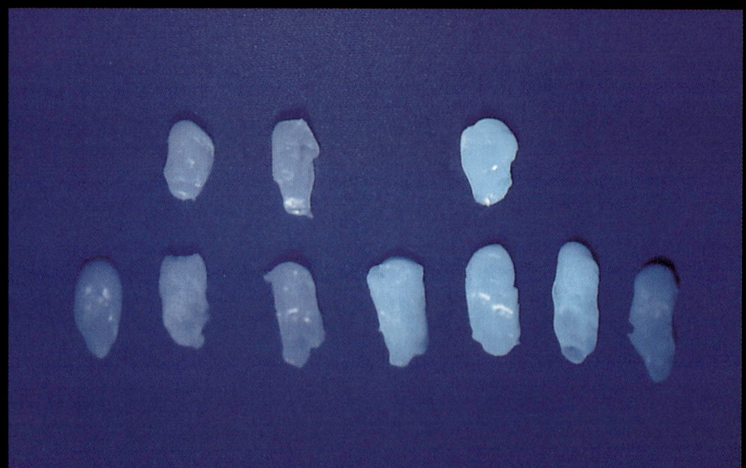
Fluorescence

Composites

Composite materials from different manufacturers in the indicated A3 colors are shown. They exhibit differences in hue, transparency and fluorescence. The decisive factor for the success of restorative treatment is not the manufacturer but rather the type of restorative material selected and the technique used to work the material.

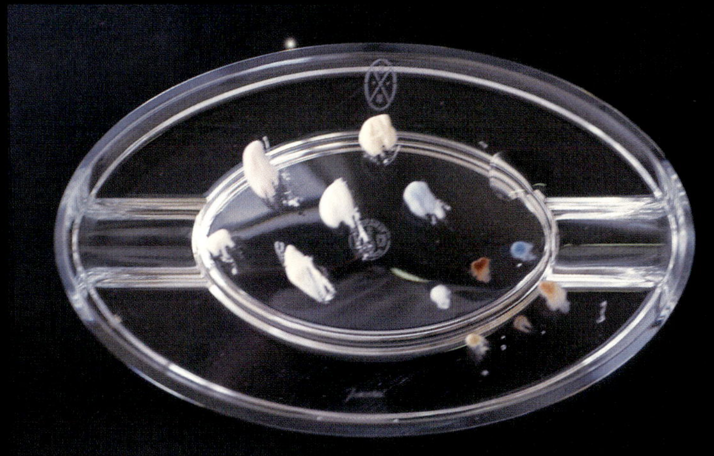

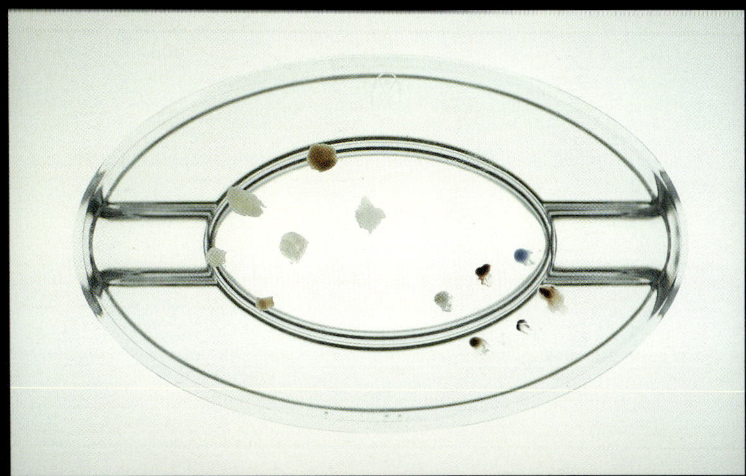

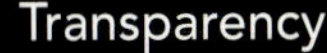

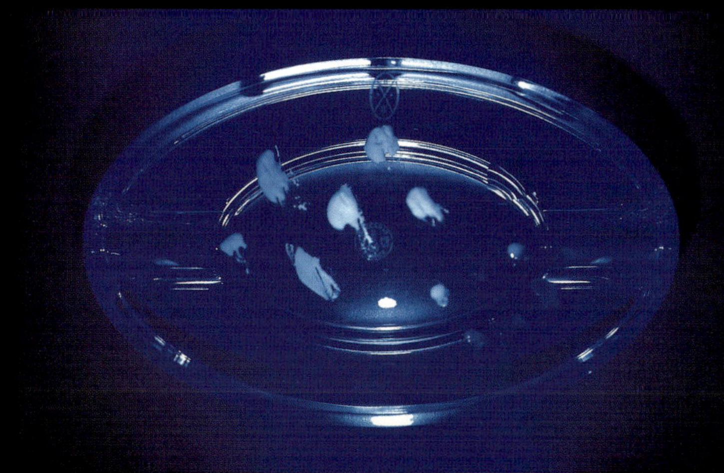

Transparency

Fluorescence

Ceramic materials

Most of the ceramic materials used in dentistry today consist of fluorescent feldspathic porcelain. Paints lacking fluorescent properties seem to disappear in infrared light (bottom right).

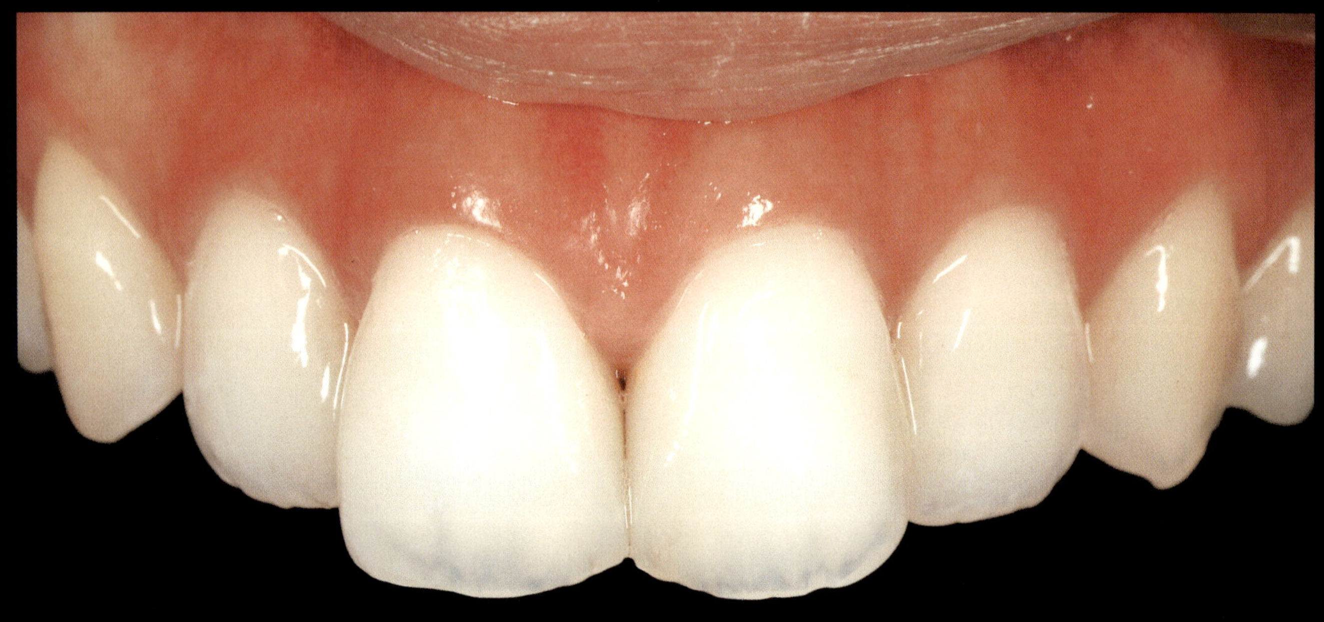

Resin composite

This photograph shows a composite restoration. Resin composite was applied to the distal part of the maxillary central incisor in layers and shaped.

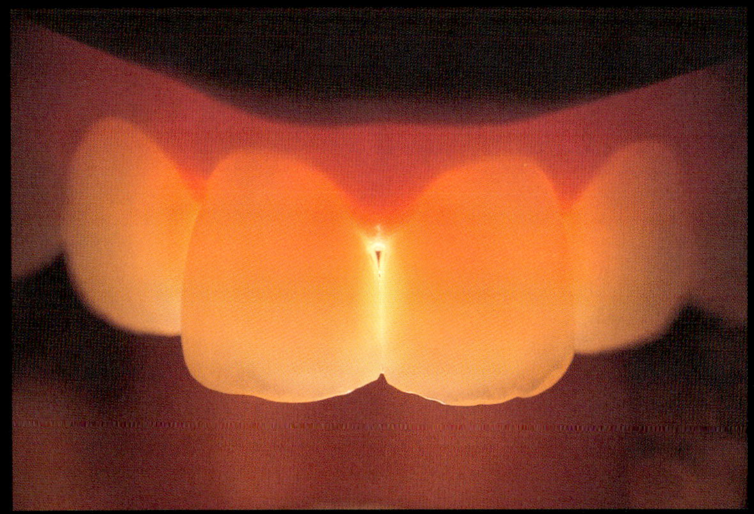

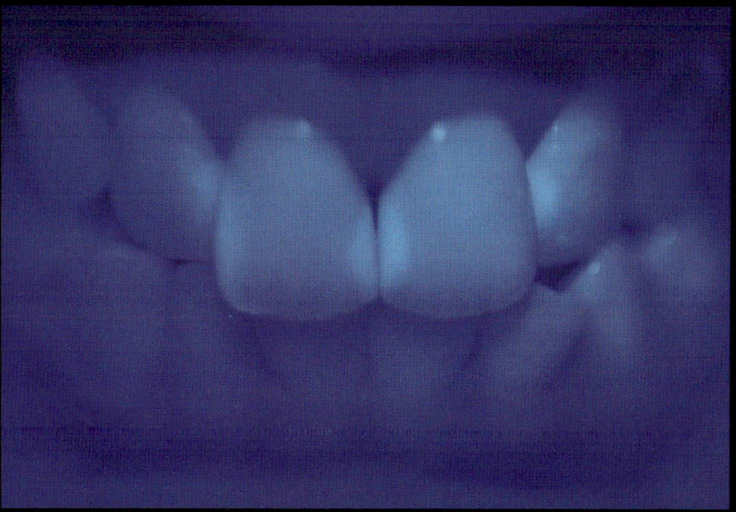

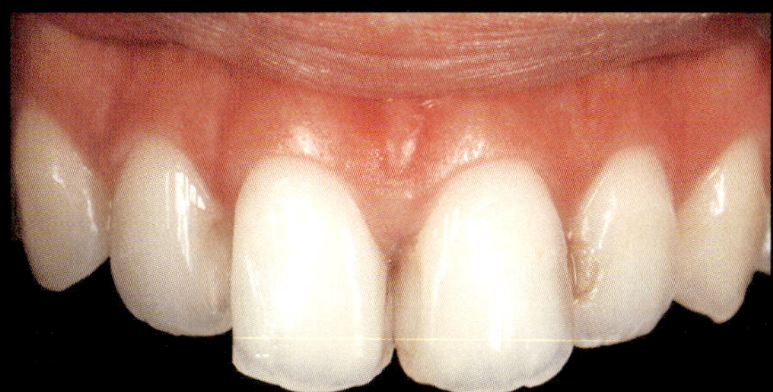

The translucency of the restoration is comparable to that of the natural teeth. In the author's opinion, the fluorescence of the composite material used here appears to be somewhat stronger than that of the teeth of Asian subjects.

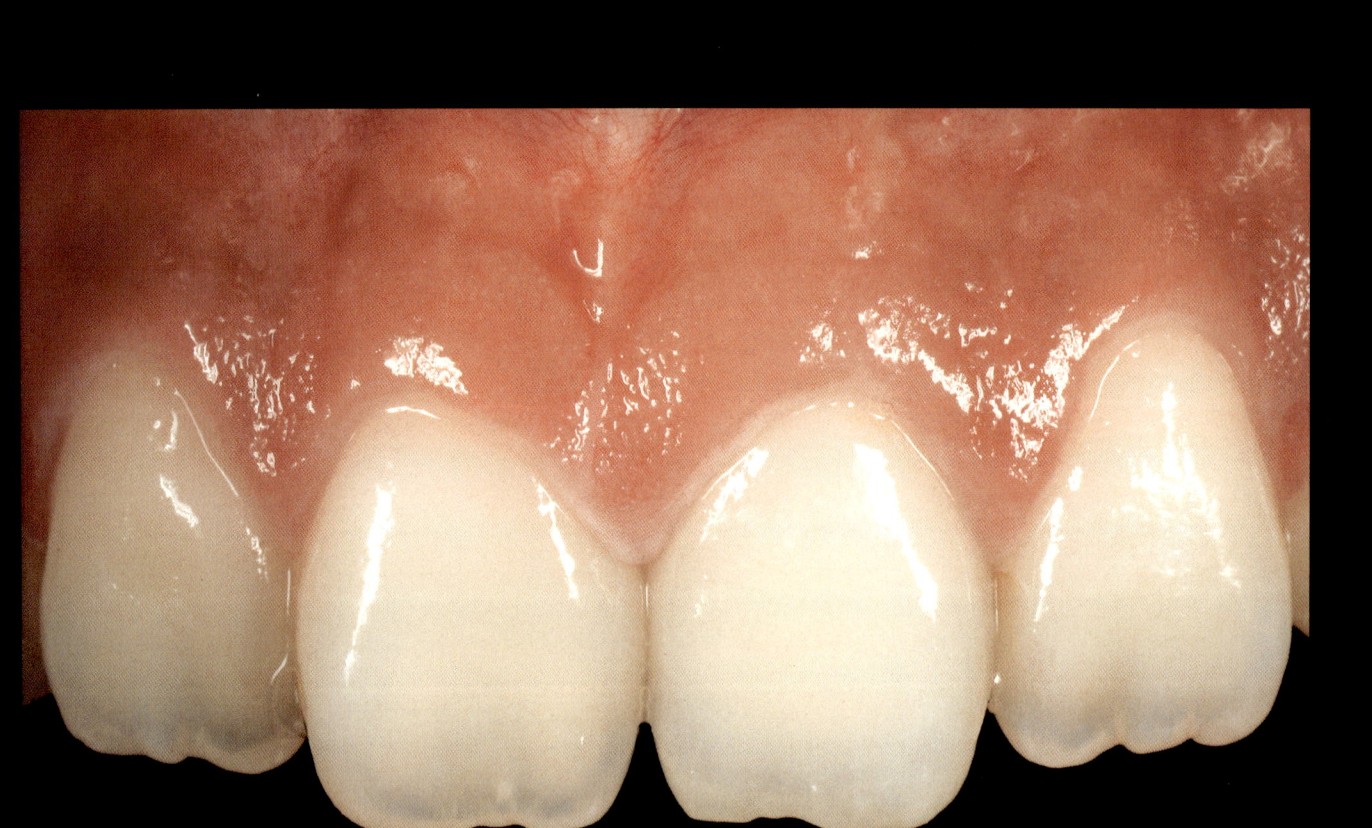

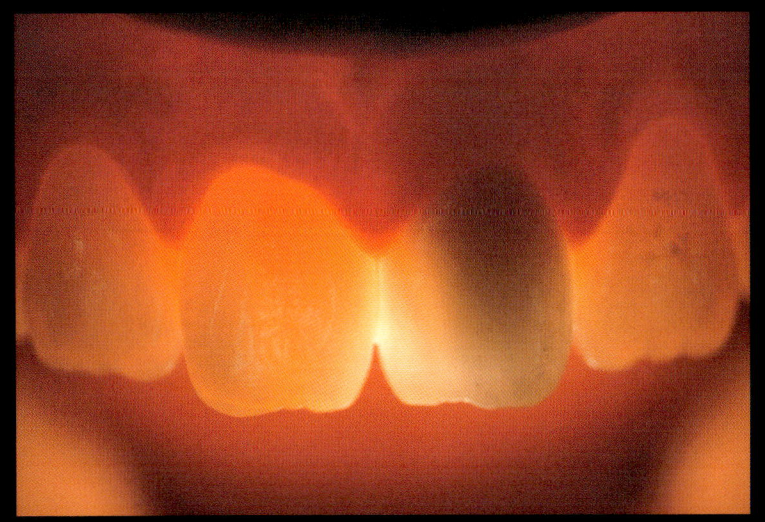

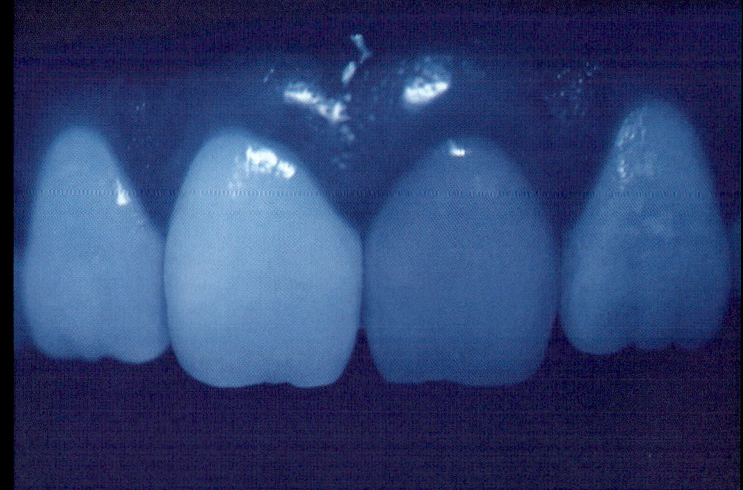

In transillumination, the cervical part of a PFM crown appears dark because light cannot shine through the metal. In infrared light, the crown virtually disappears from sight in spite of the fact that the ceramic material is fluorescent. The lack of translucency and fluorescence sometimes plays tricks on the eyes in alternating light conditions.

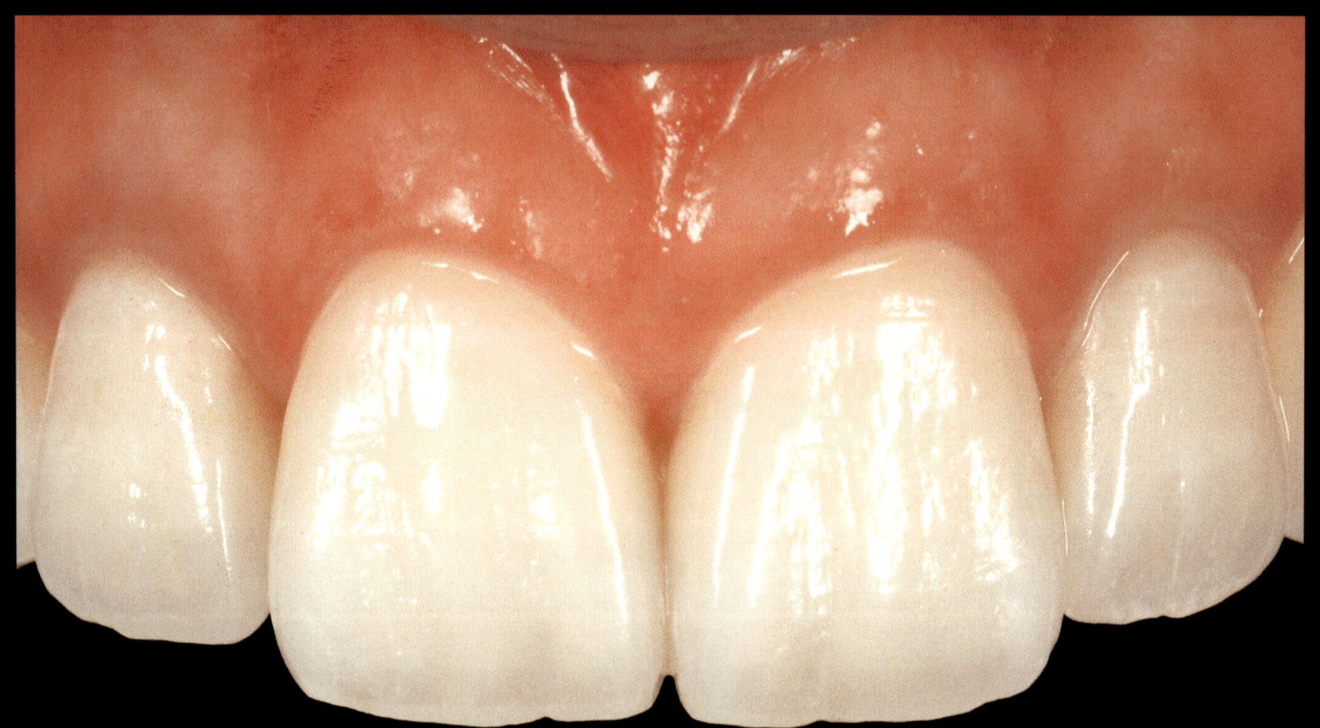

Porcelain veneers

The mechanical and optical properties of feldspathic porcelain are very similar to those of the natural tooth enamel.

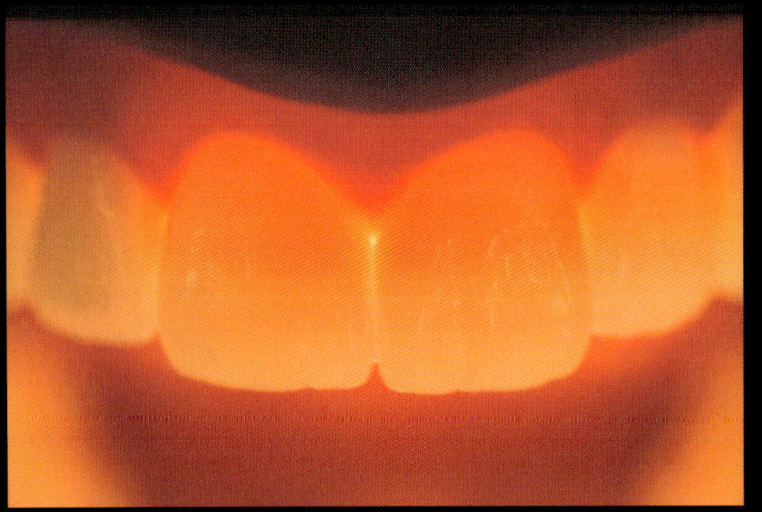

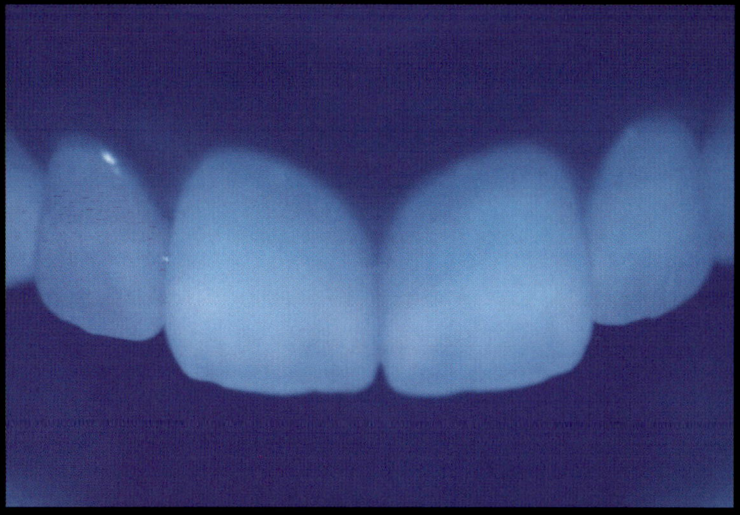

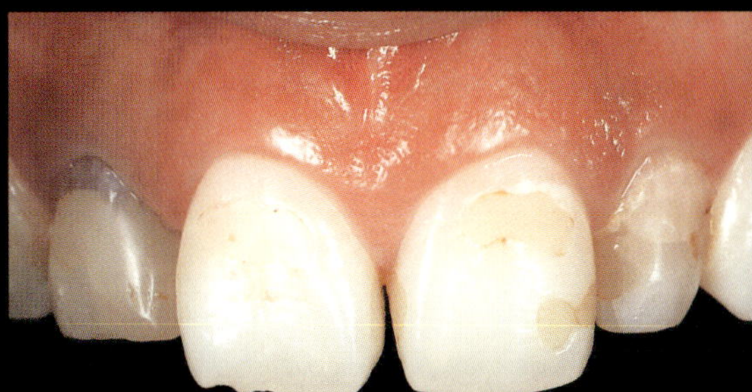

Porcelain veneer restorations have a natural appearance that very closely resembles that of natural teeth in different lighting conditions. Porcelain restorations are unsurpassed by other restorative options in cases in which tooth enamel is still present.

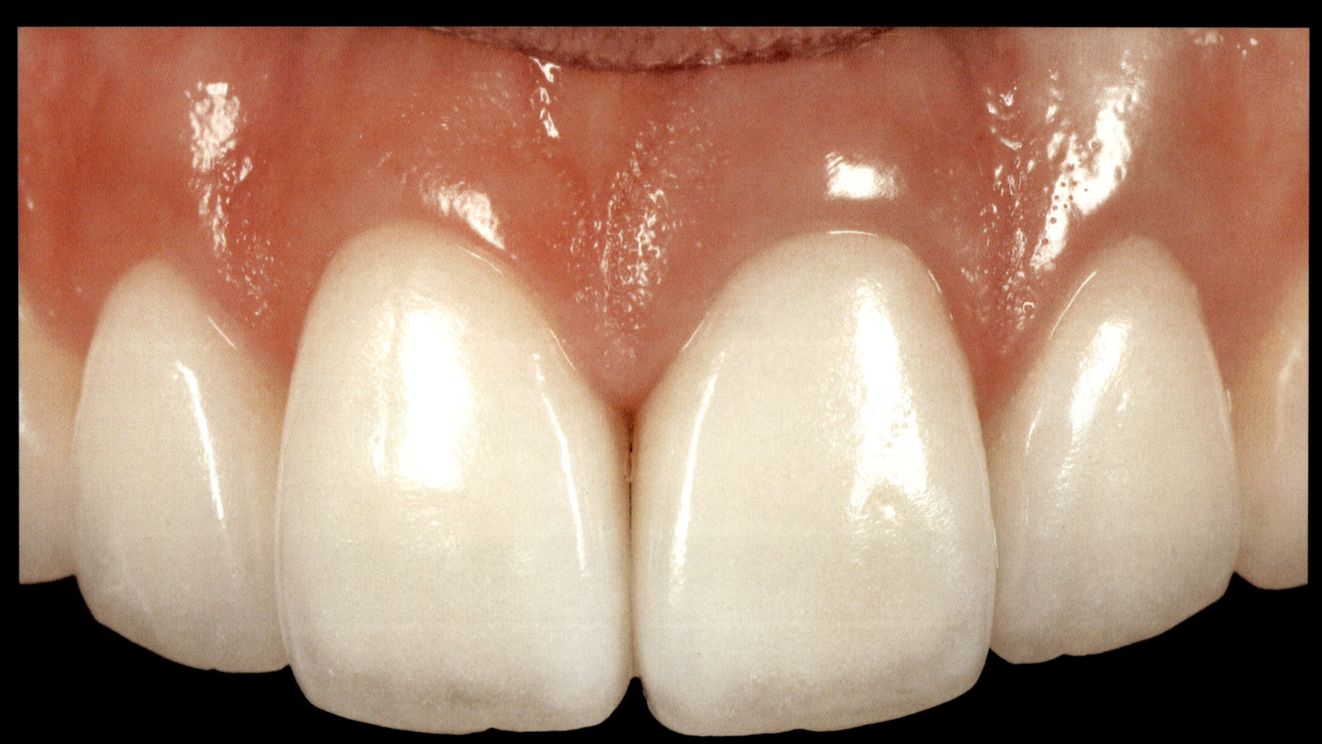

IPS Empress2

All-ceramic crowns made of ceramic material with a crystalline content (lithium disilicate crystals, $LiO_2 \cdot 2SiO_2$).

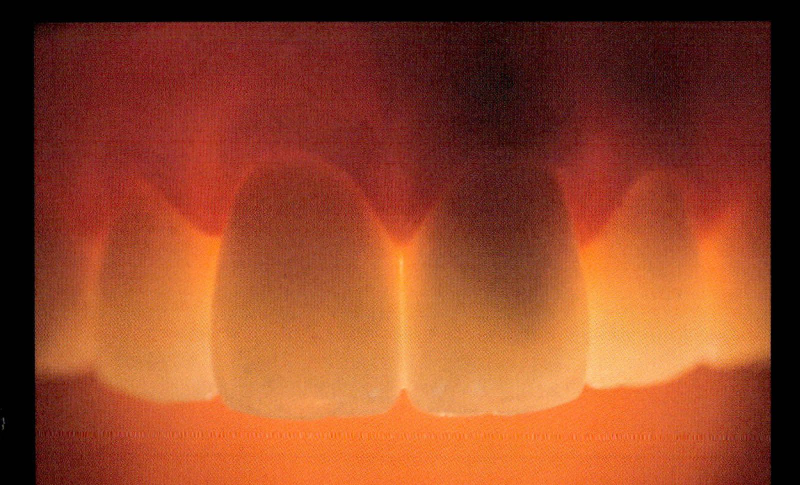

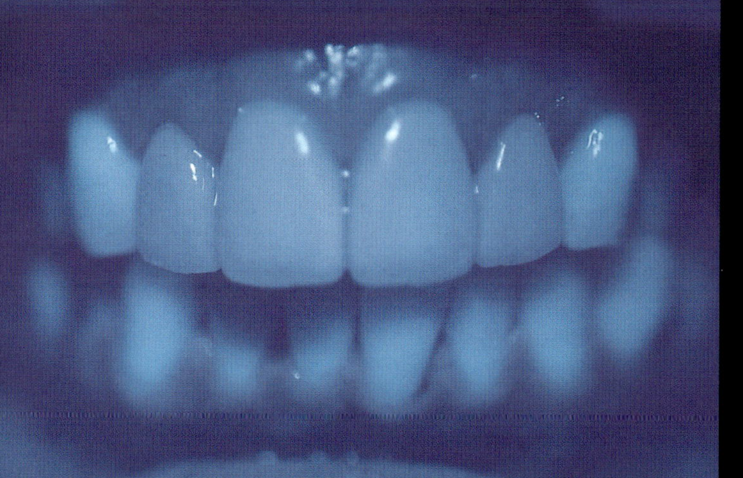

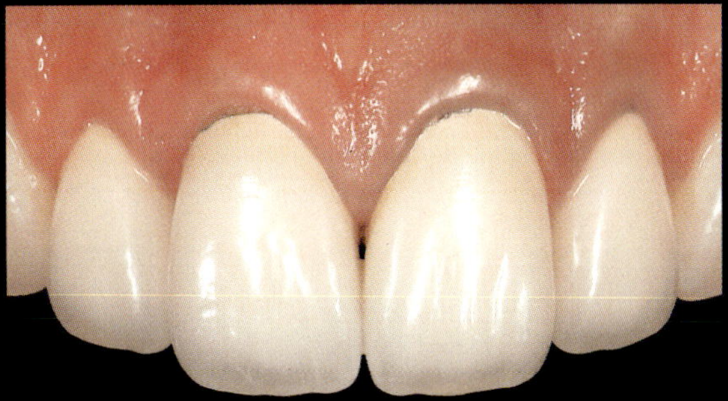

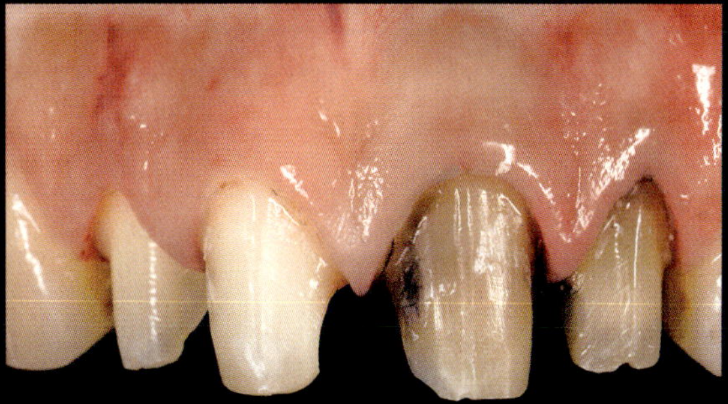

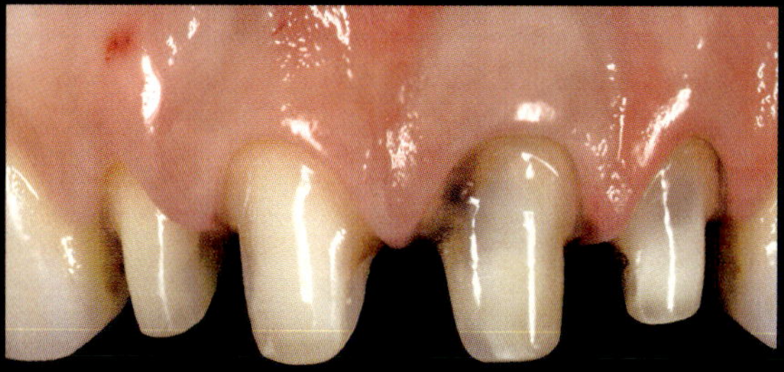

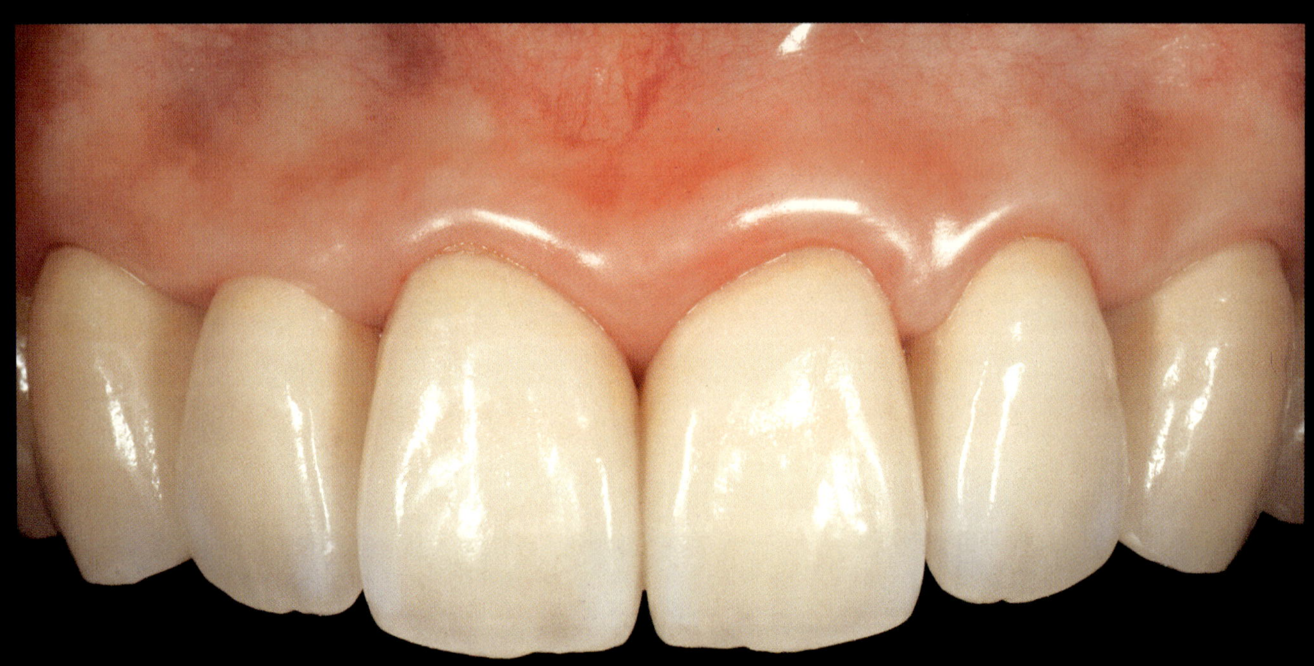

Procera 0.6 mm

All-ceramic crowns made of aluminum oxide (Al_2O_3)

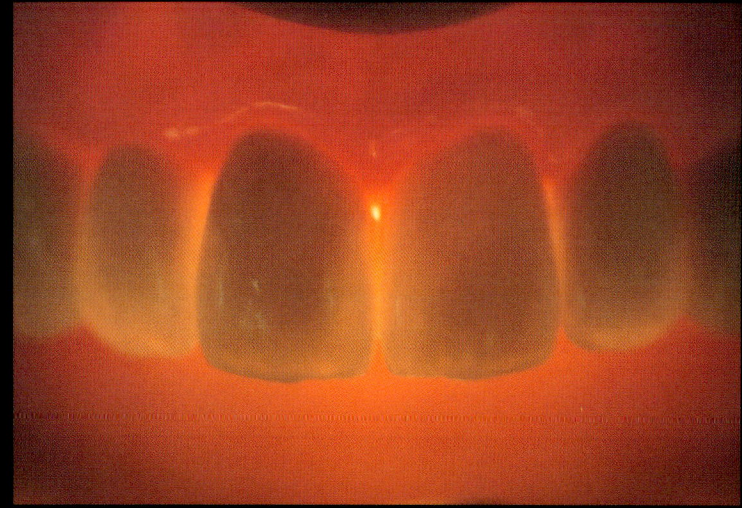

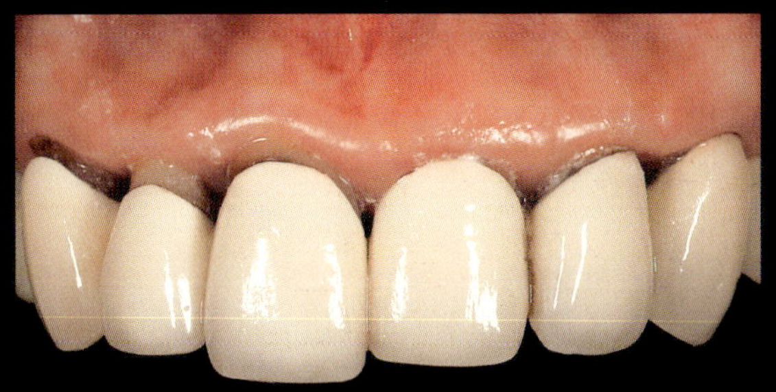

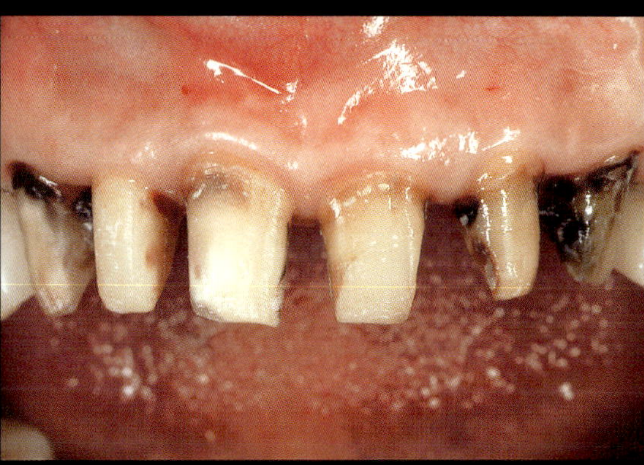

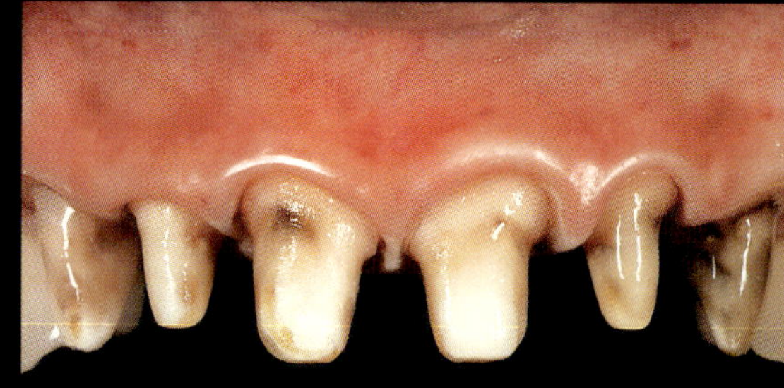

Since all of the abutment teeth were vital teeth, it was not possible to match the shades of the teeth by bleaching. In order to mask the shade differences, less translucent Procera 0.6 was used as the cap material. With this type of material, the cervical zone does not become as dark as in restorations with metal substructures.

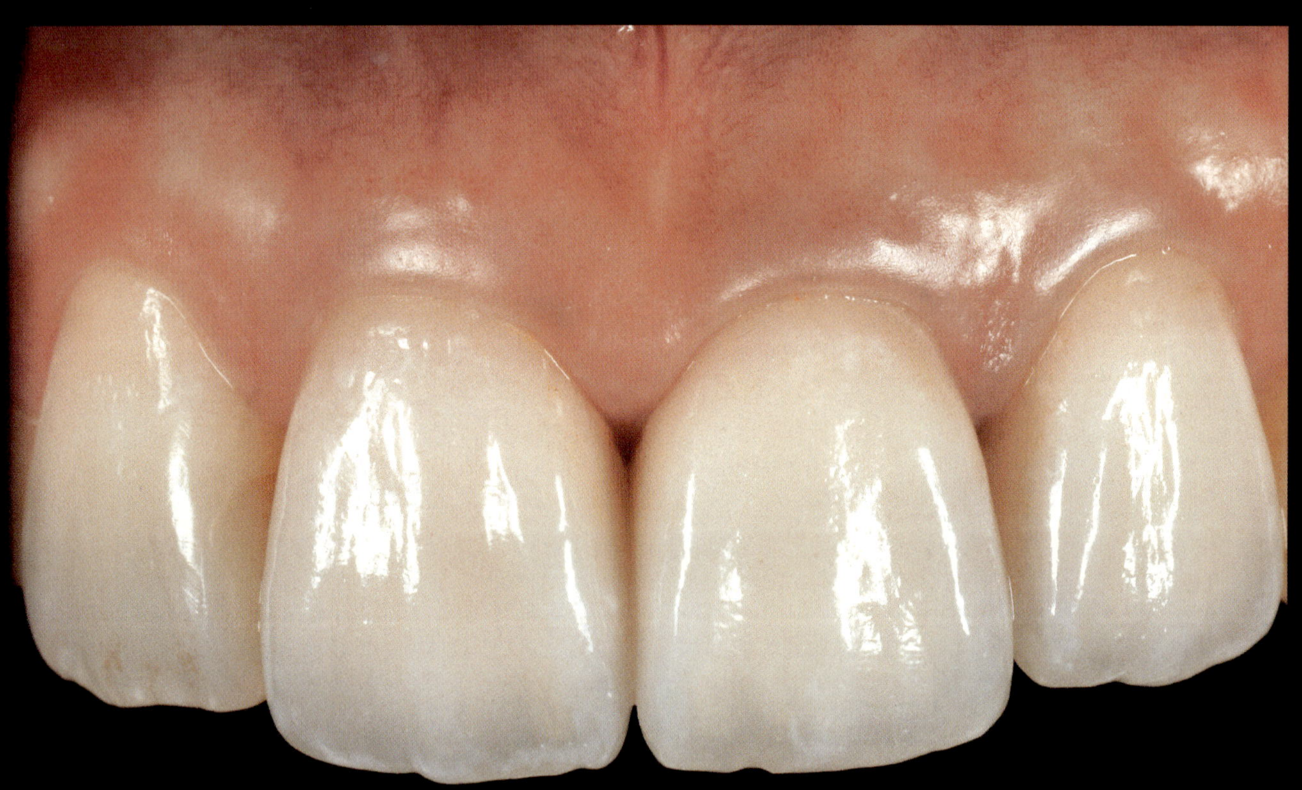

Procera 0.4 mm

All-ceramic crowns made of aluminum oxide (Al_20_3).

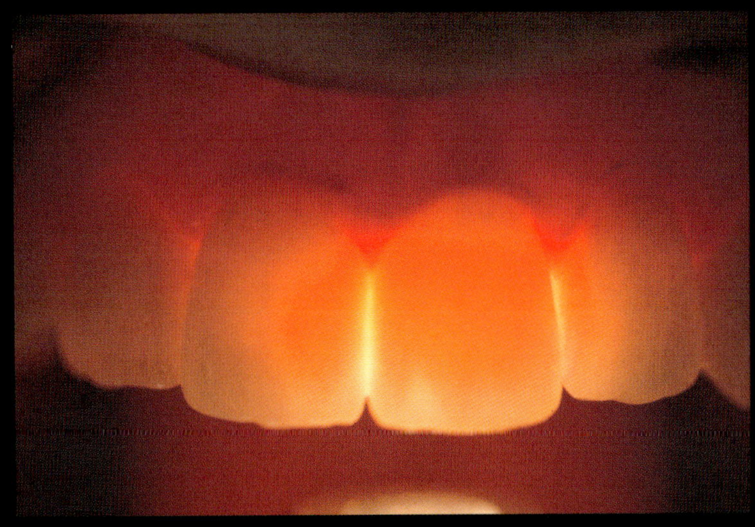

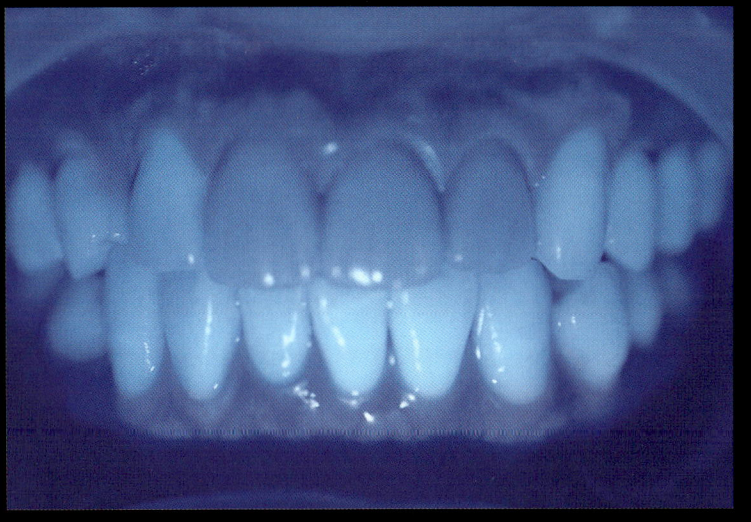

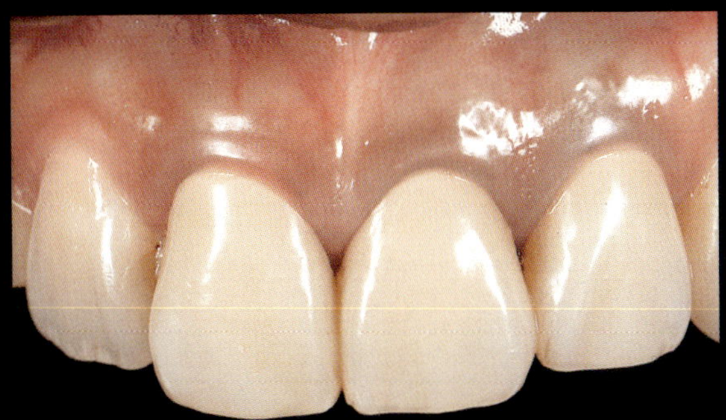

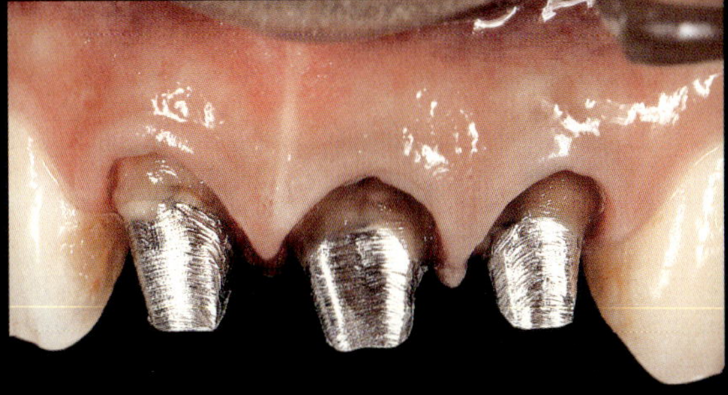

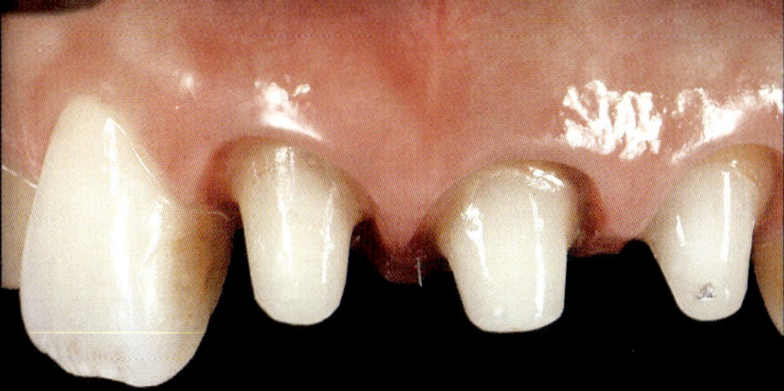

The main concern here was to improve the darkness of the cervical zone. The metal posts were therefore replaced with glass fiber posts and composite cores. Aluminum oxide restorations feature very high translucency that is almost identical to that of the natural healthy teeth. The degree of fluorescence is not as low as that of metal, but still very low.

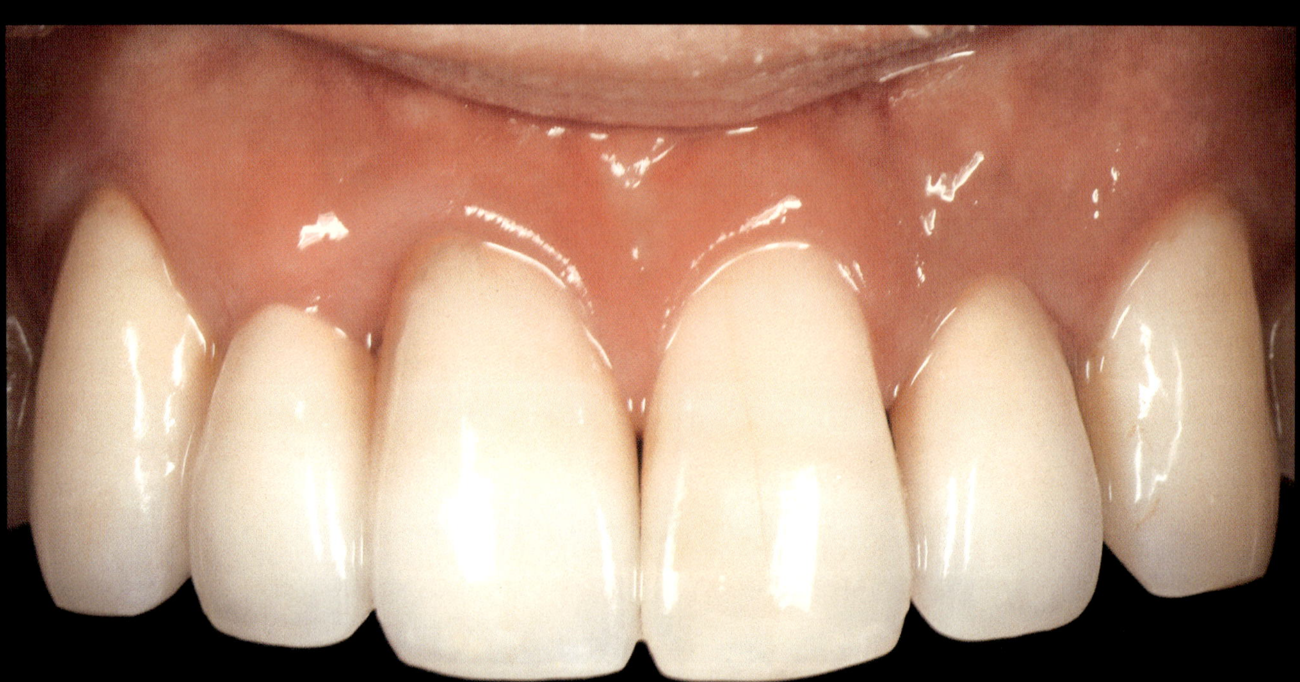

In-Ceram

All-ceramic crowns made of crystalline aluminum oxide (Al_2O_3).

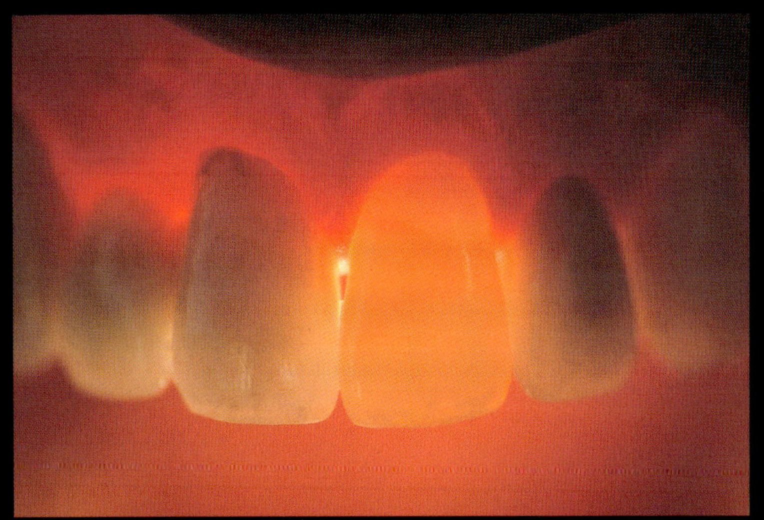
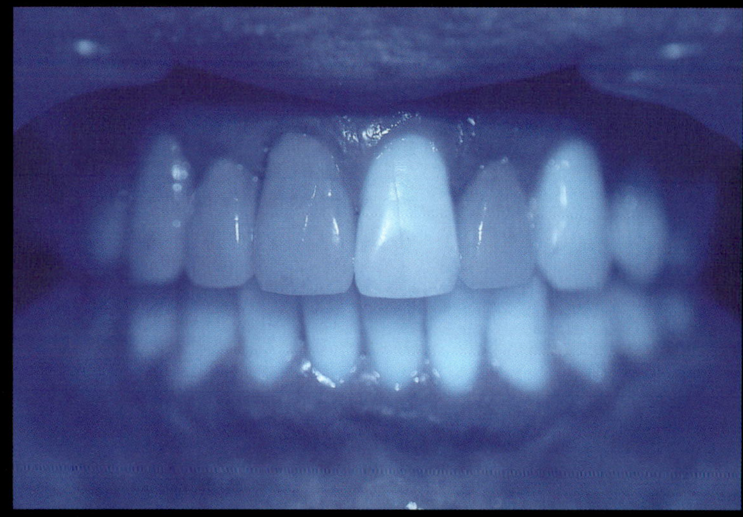
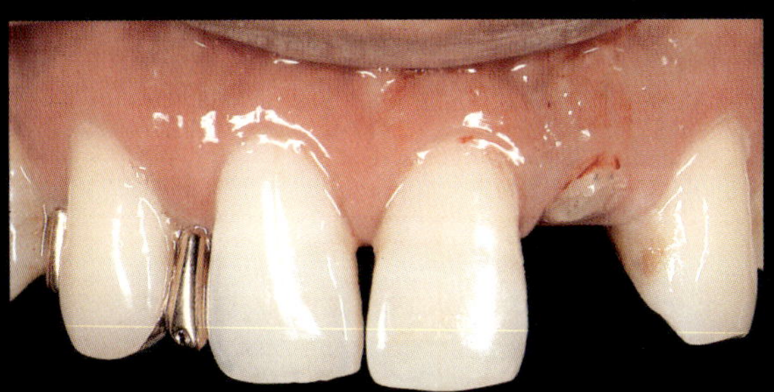
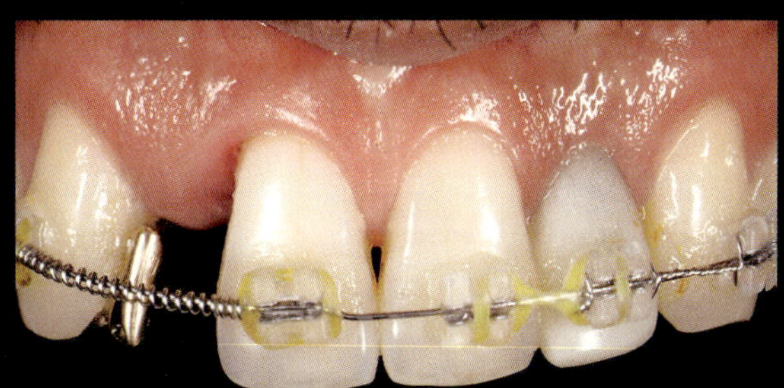
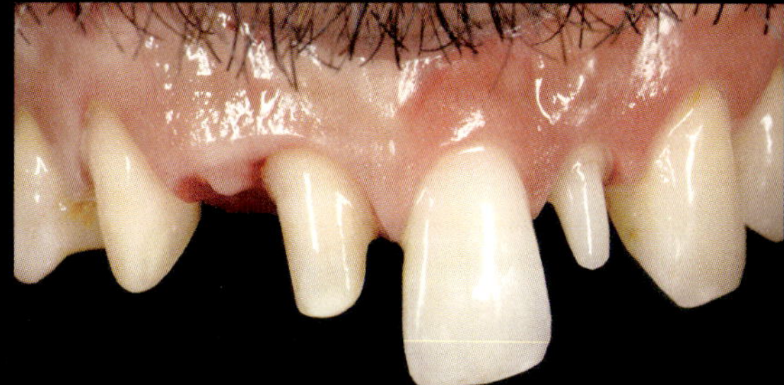

Although the translucency of In-Ceram is lower than that of Procera, another aluminum oxide ceramic, the cervical zone is not as dark as that of metal. Fluorescence of In-Ceram is low and comparable to that of metal.

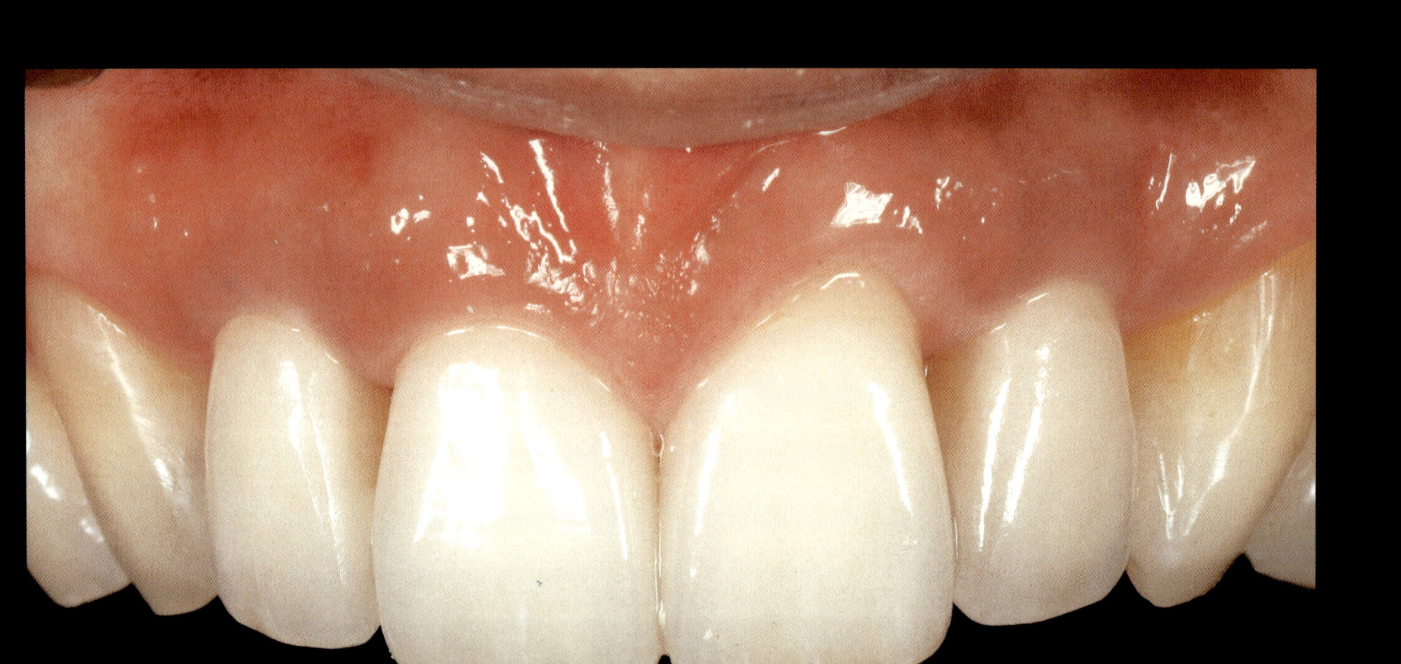

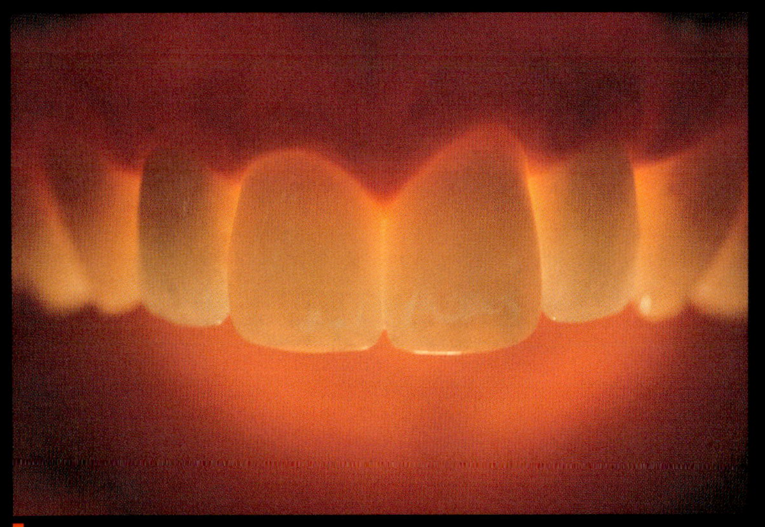

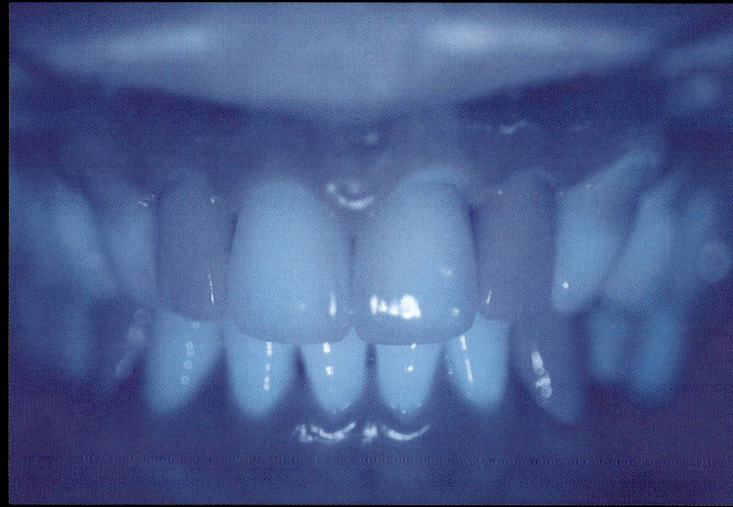

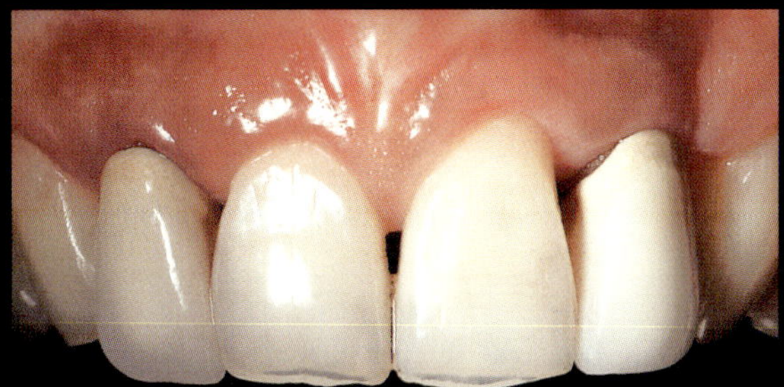

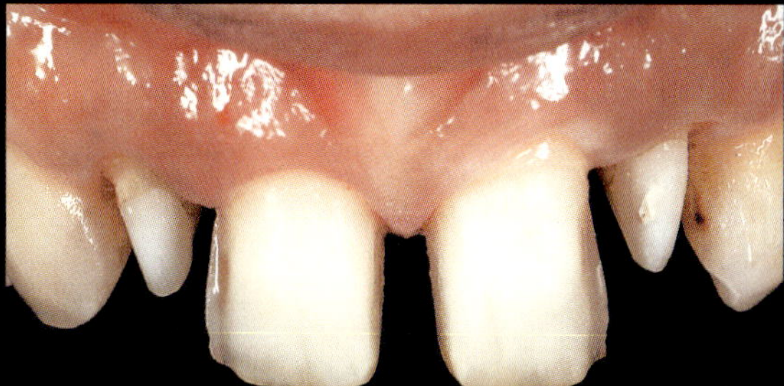

In-Ceram Spinell was used to fabricate the crowns on teeth 12 and 22. This material has high translucency. However, its fluorescence is not very different from that of metal (the restorations on teeth 44 and 33 are porcelain-fused-to-metal crowns).

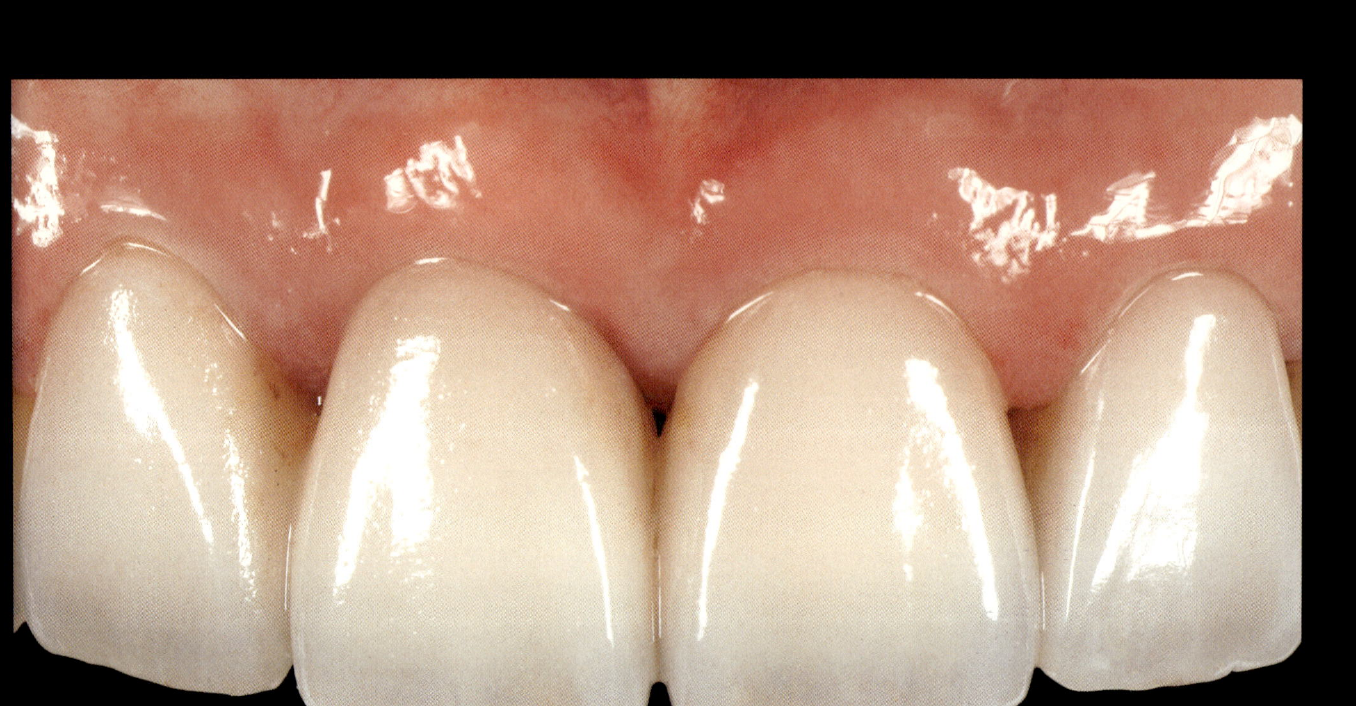

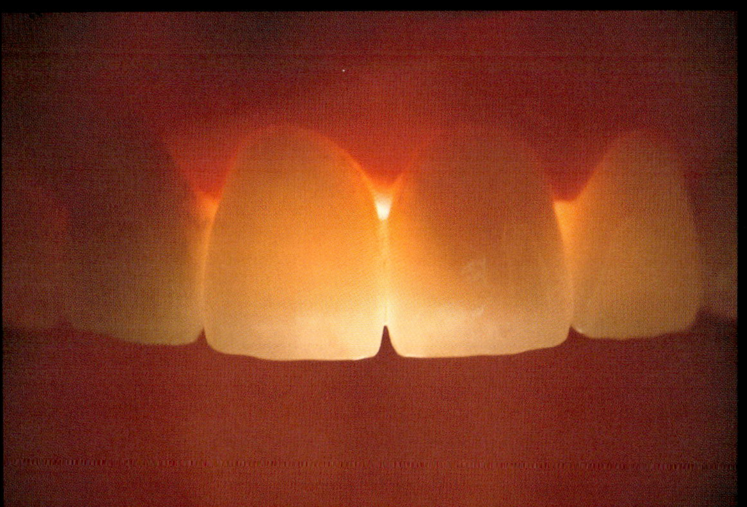

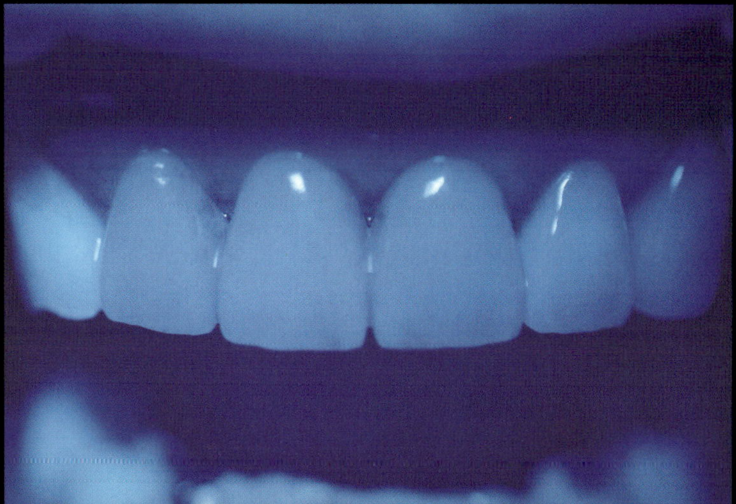

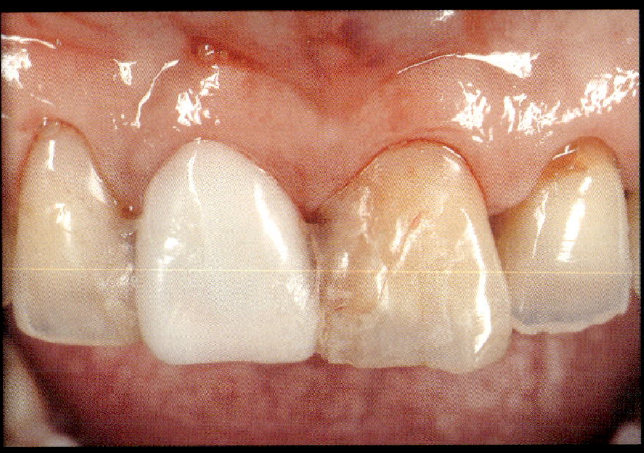

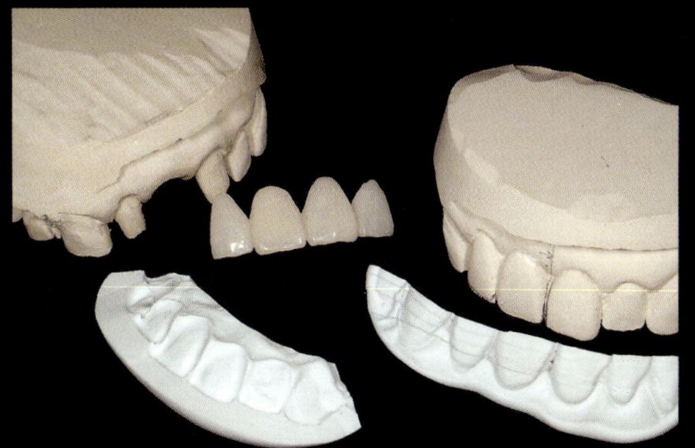

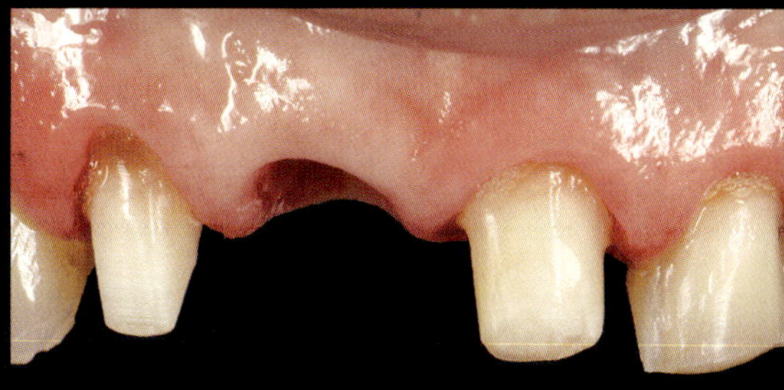

Improvement of transparency was achieved by reducing the layer thickness of the translucent zirconium dioxide material to 0.3 mm. Although the fluorescence of Lava is not as low as that of metal, it is not very high (tooth 13 is a natural tooth).

Porcelain-fused-to-metal crown
with a cast metal post and core

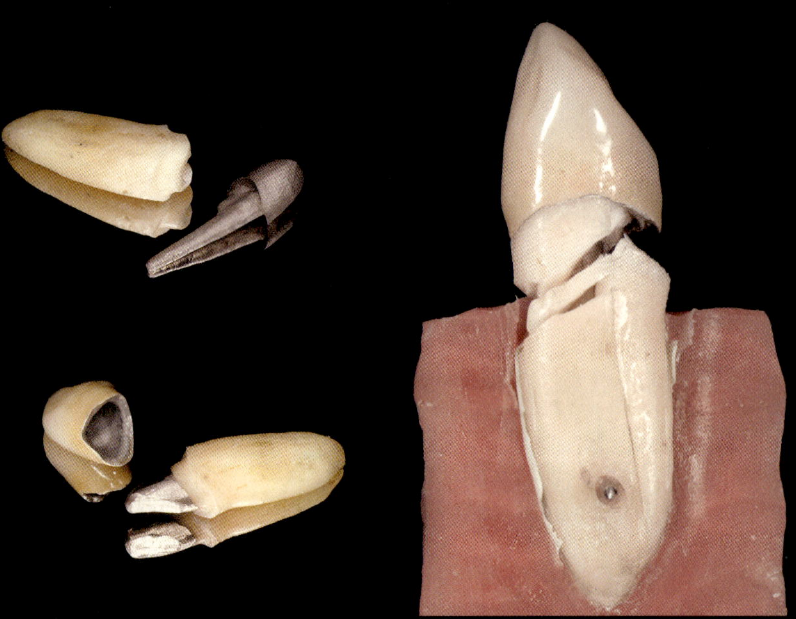

All-ceramic crown (Al_2O_3)
with a glass fiber/composite post and core

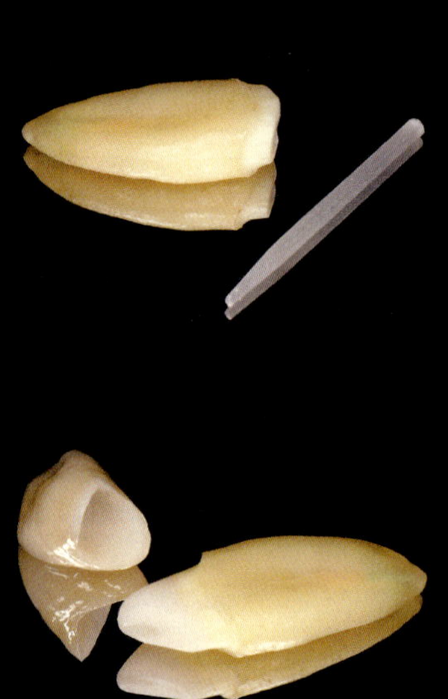

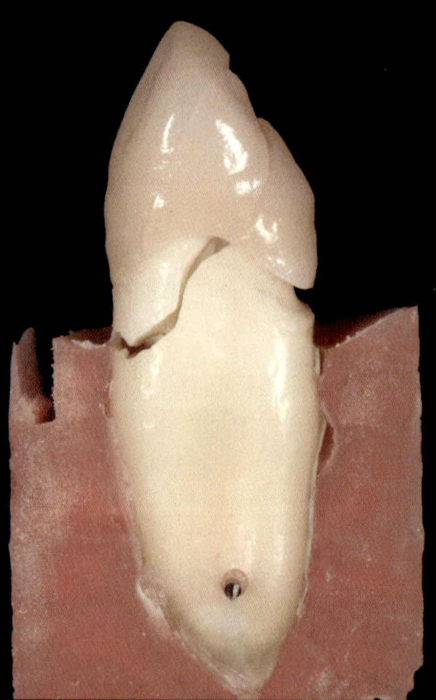

Catastrophic Failure

The strength and fracture toughness of glass fiber/composite post-and-core restorations is virtually identical to that of conventional metal post and core restorations. In fact, vertical fractures that extend to the tooth root and make retreatment impossible are more frequently observed with cast metal post and core restorations. Higher strength and toughness do not necessarily mean better.

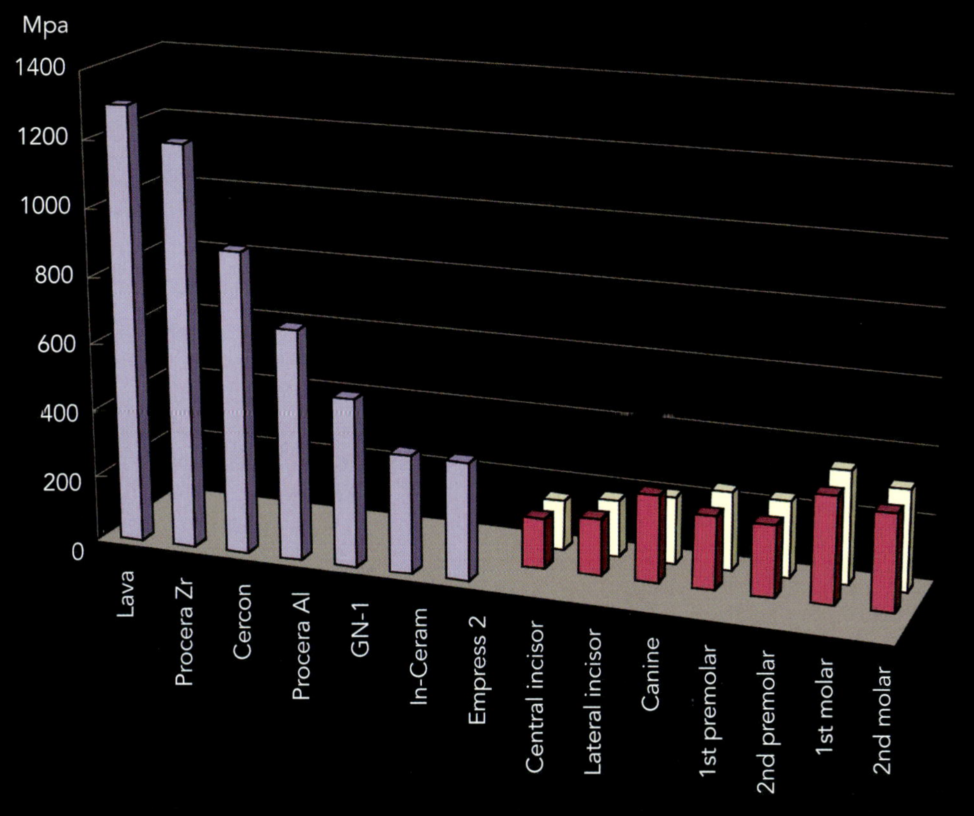

Biaxial flexural strength

The appropriateness of a given ceramic material is determined by the forces exerted on the tooth and the strength of the respective material.
It is important to know that most all-ceramic crowns lose up to half of their original strength after placement in the mouth of the patient.

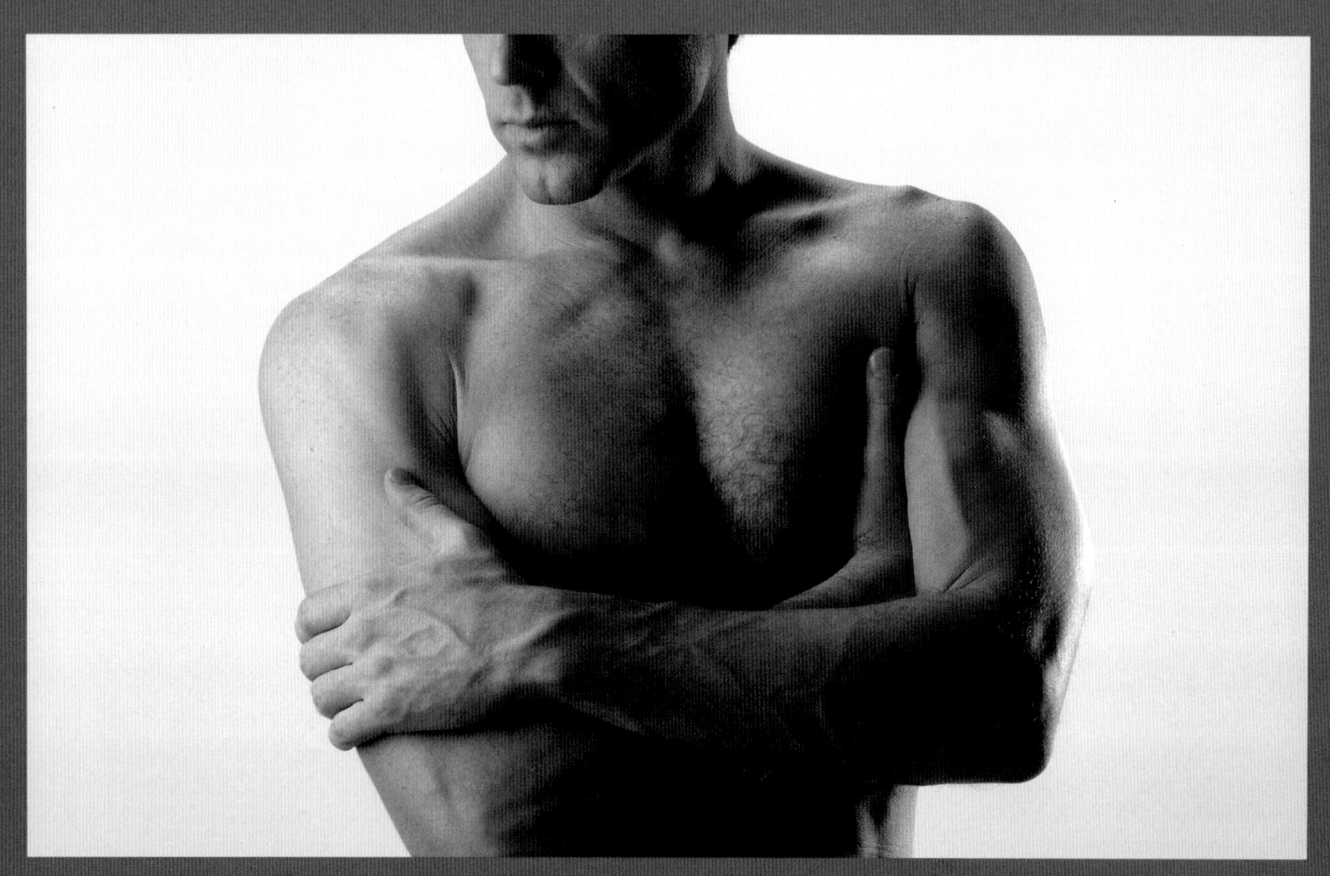

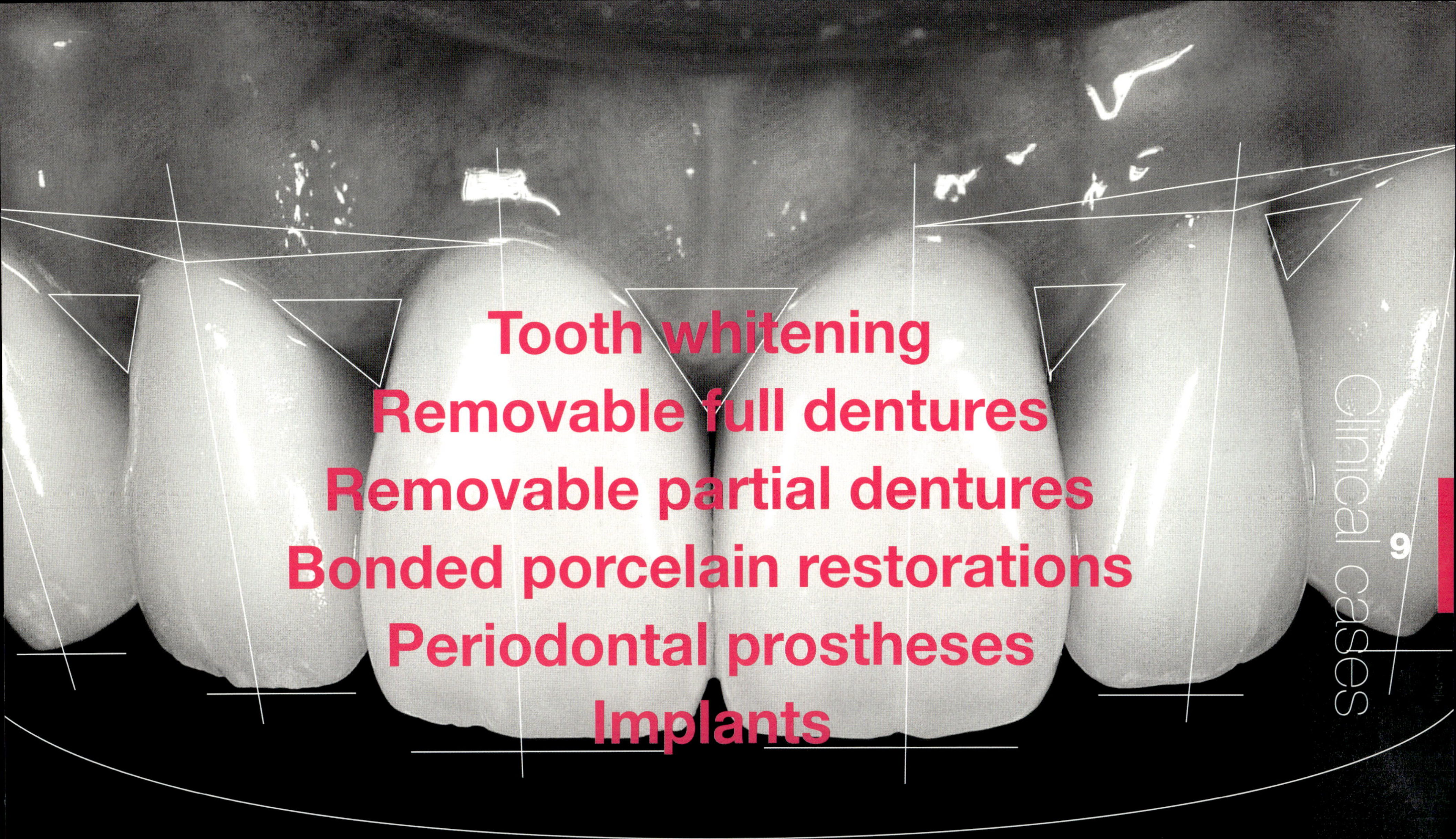
Tooth whitening
Removable full dentures
Removable partial dentures
Bonded porcelain restorations
Periodontal prostheses
Implants
Clinical cases
9

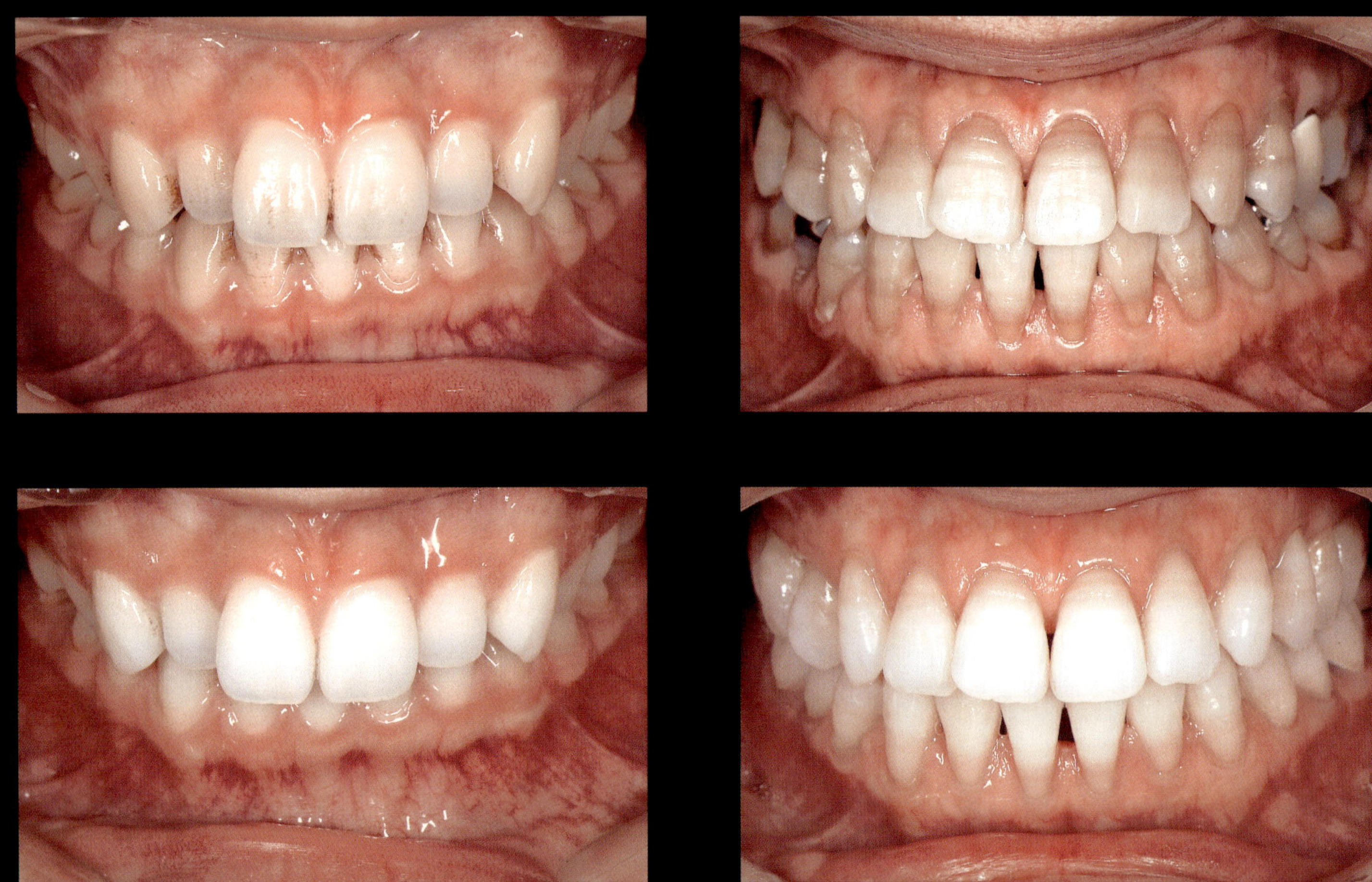

Tooth whitening

Dentists generally prefer ivory-colored teeth, whereas most patients want to have white teeth. Therefore, one of the tasks of the dentist is to provide risk-free tooth whitening methods for the patients.

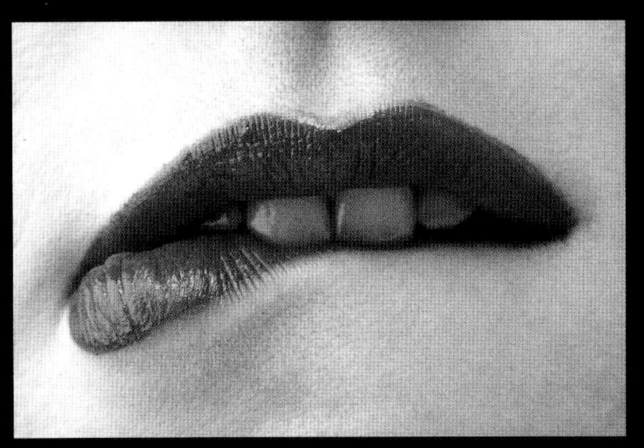
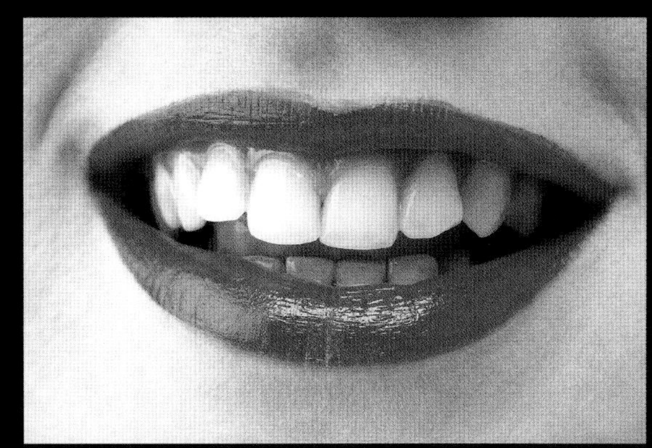
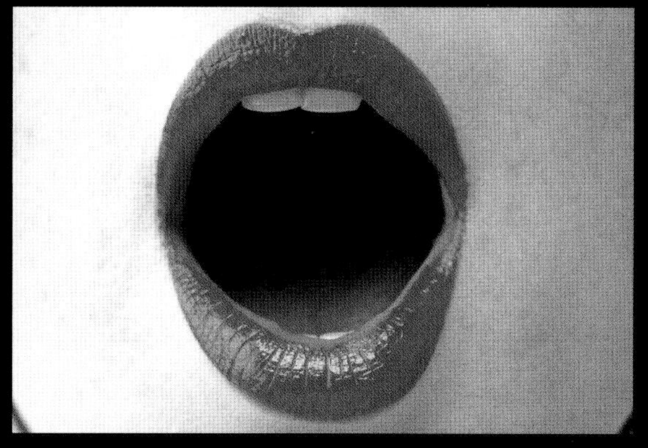
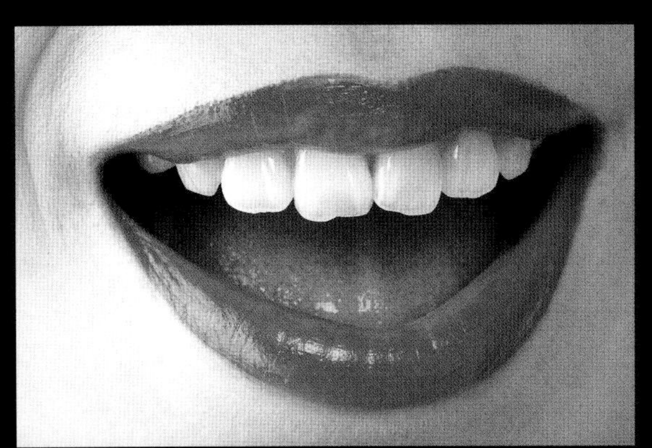
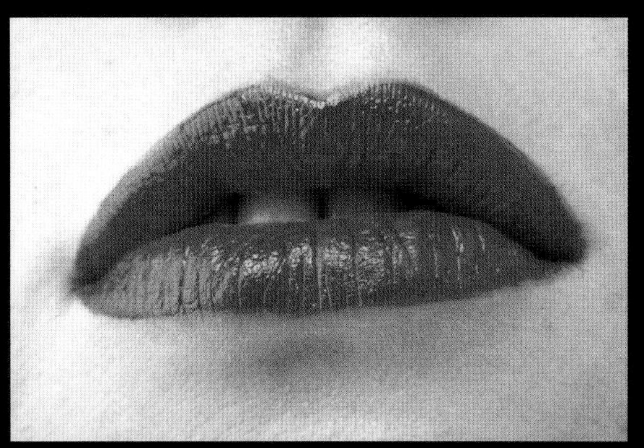
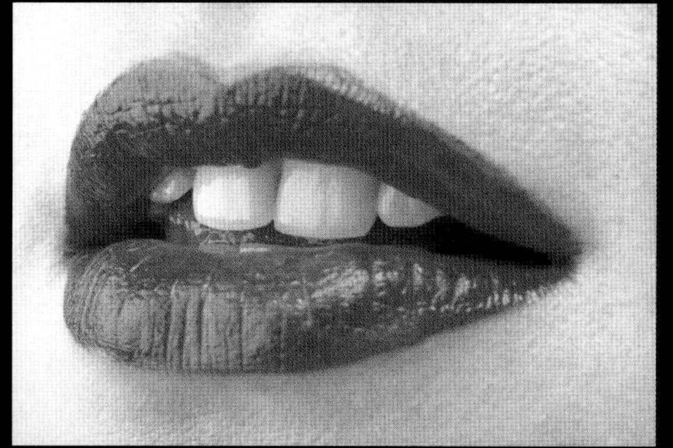

Having white teeth is a top priority for many patients.

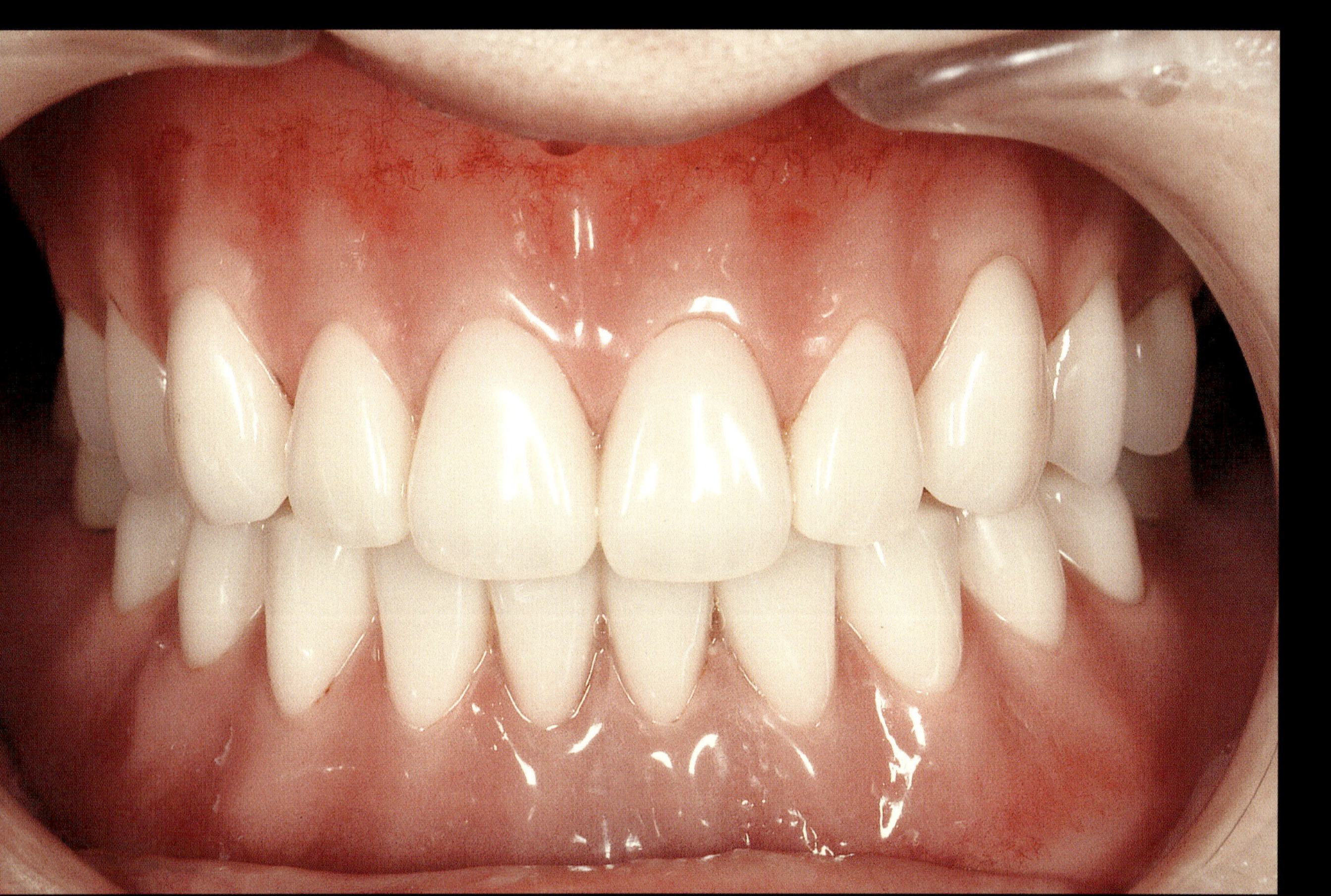

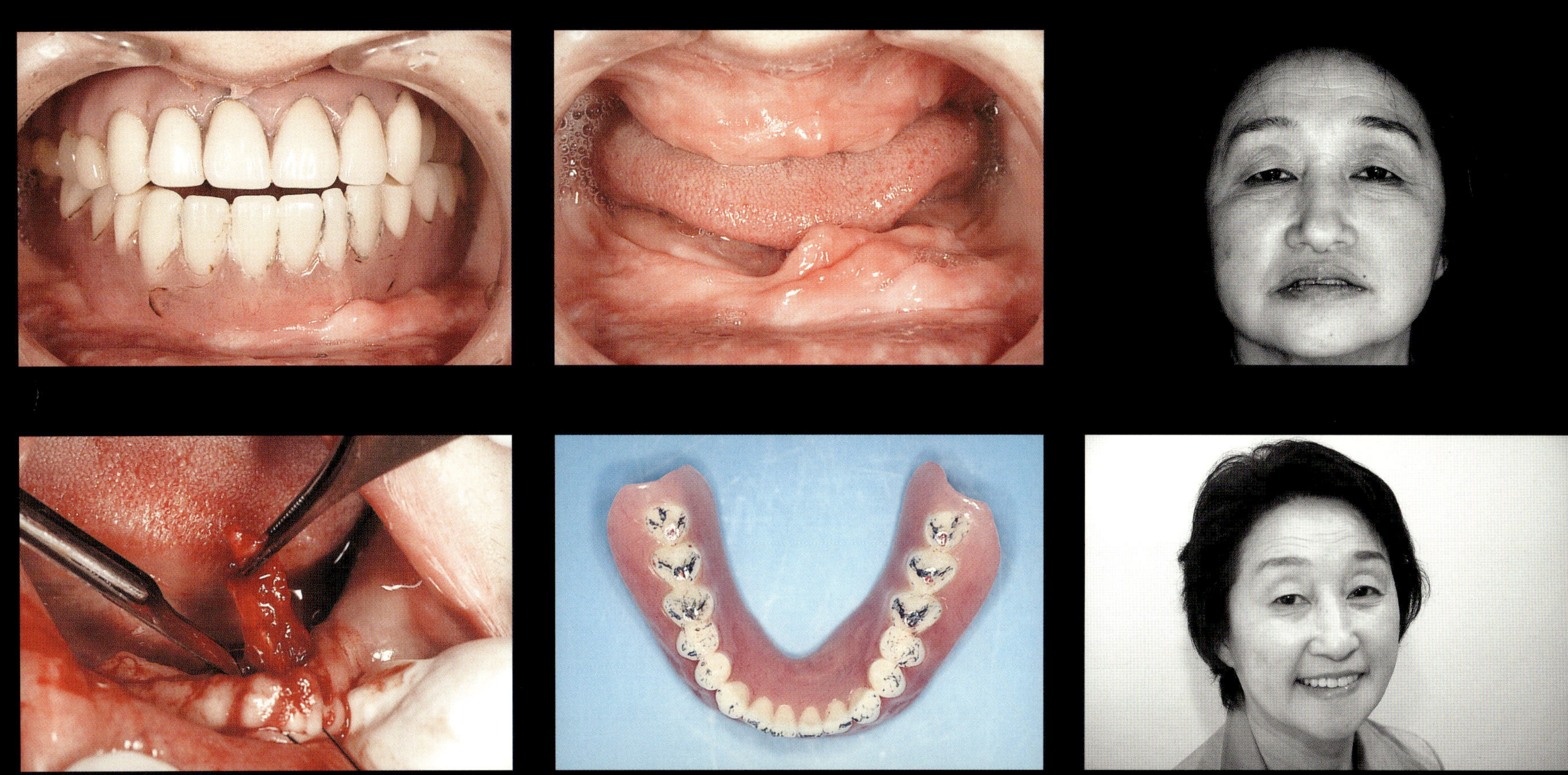

Removable full dentures

Any excess tissue must be surgically removed. Bilaterally balanced occlusion is the preferred occlusal concept for removable full dentures. Removable full dentures can change the esthetics of a patient's physiognomy very quickly.

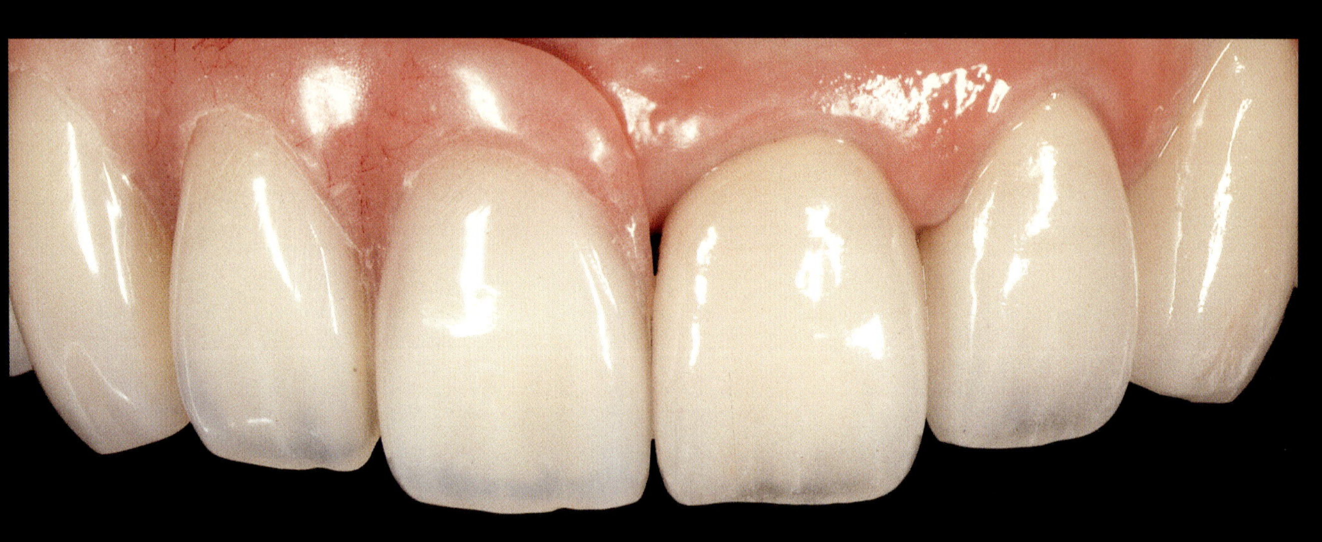

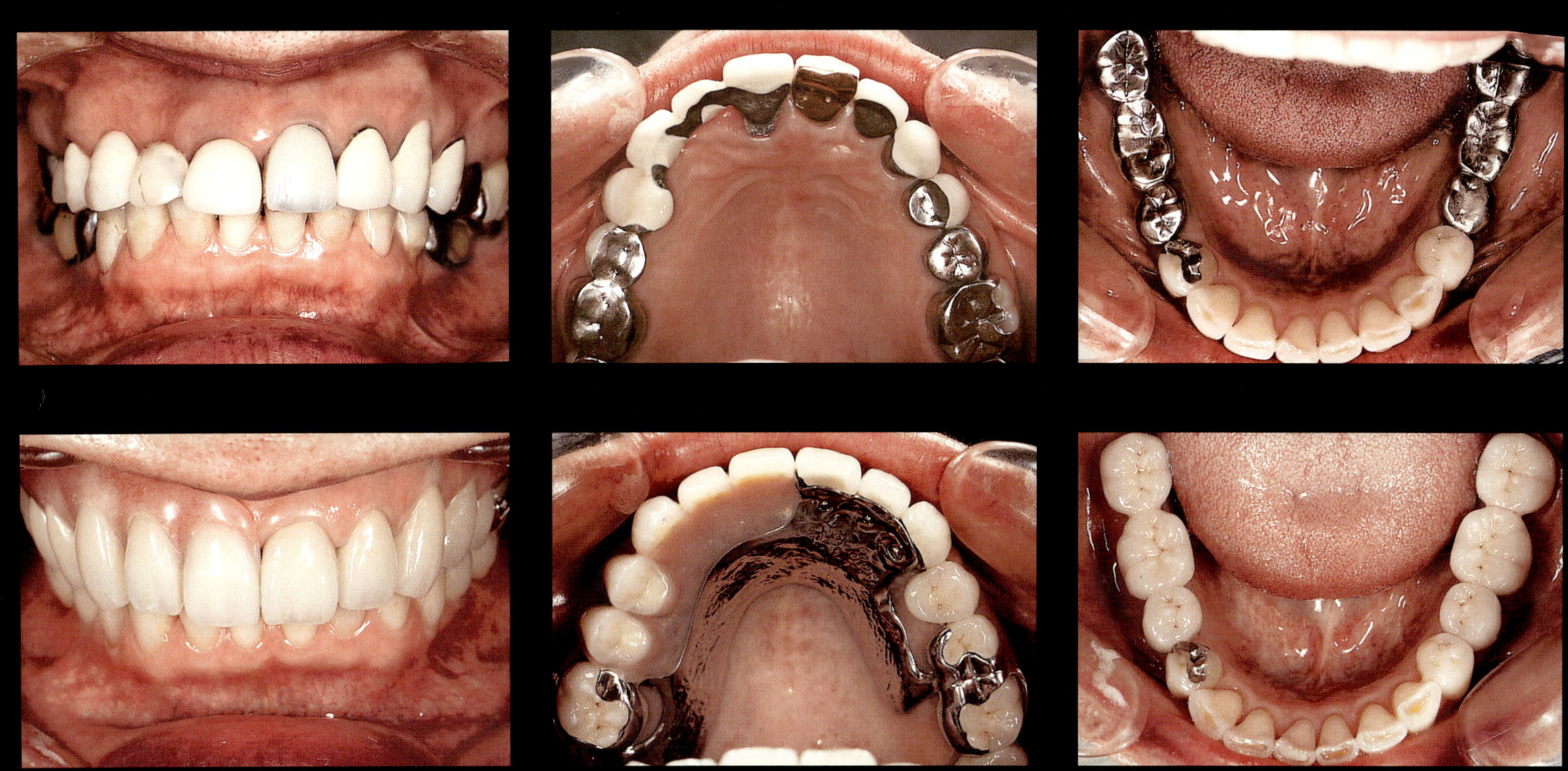

Removable partial dentures

The most important structural elements of removable partial dentures are the retainer and the guide plate. Occlusal concepts for removable partial dentures vary and are determined based on the remaining dentition.

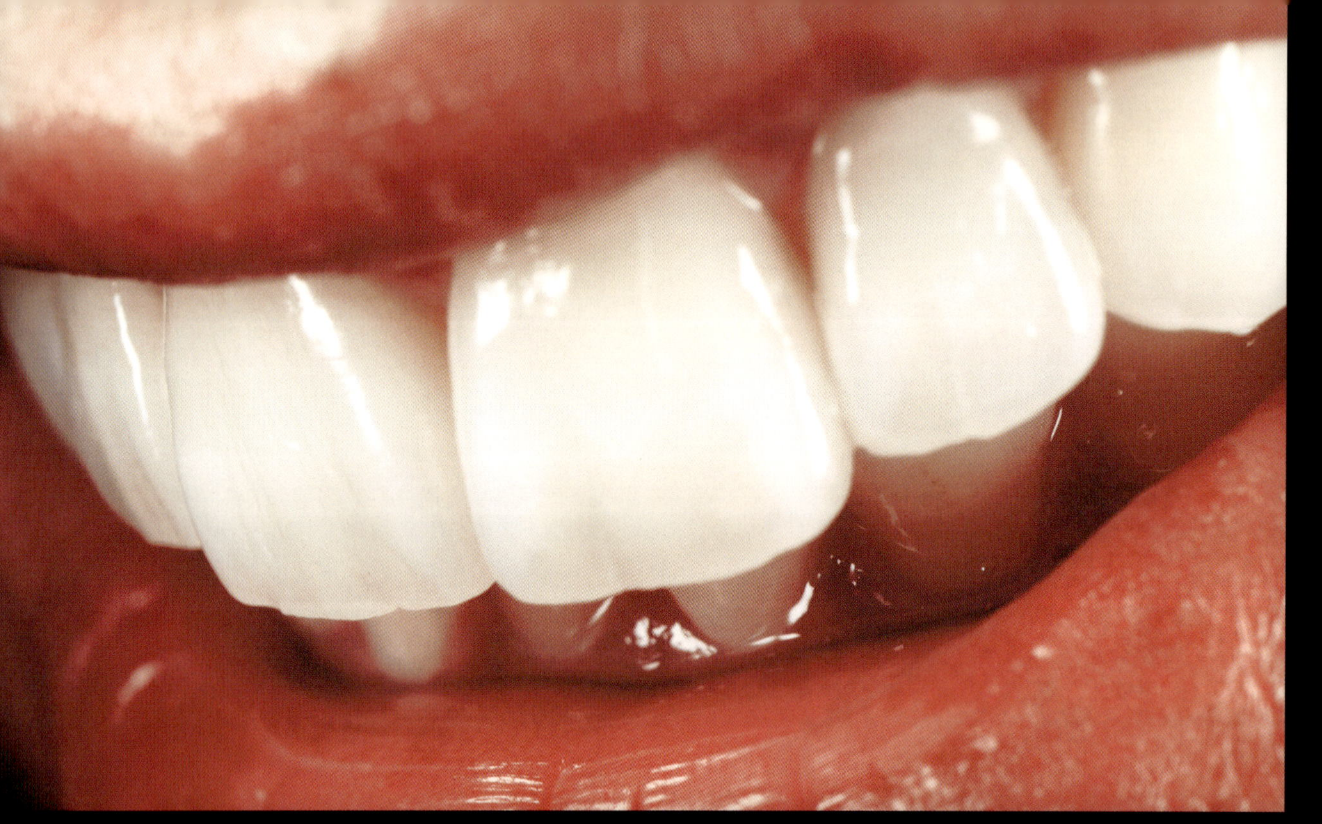

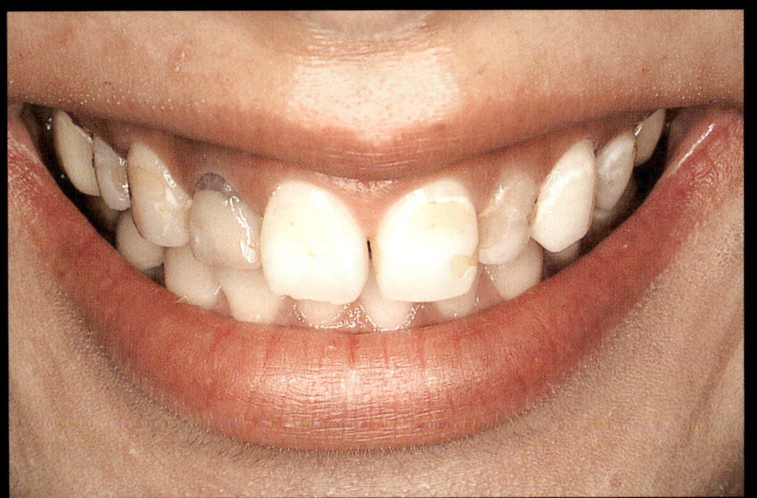

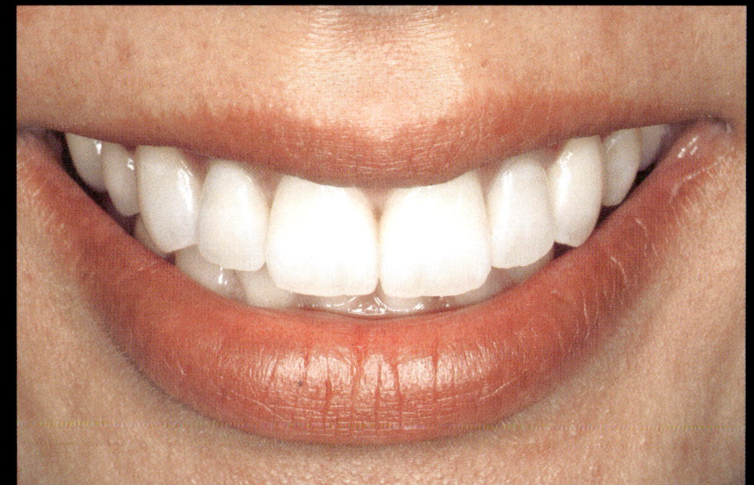

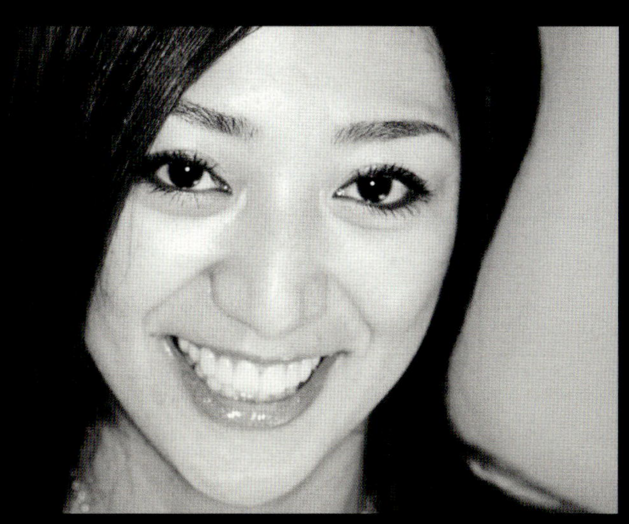

Bonded porcelain restorations

The mechanical and optical properties of feldspathic porcelain materials are very similar to those of the natural teeth. Bonded porcelain restorations in which feldspathic porcelain materials are bonded directly to the teeth are currently the best restorative option in cases in which tooth enamel is still present.

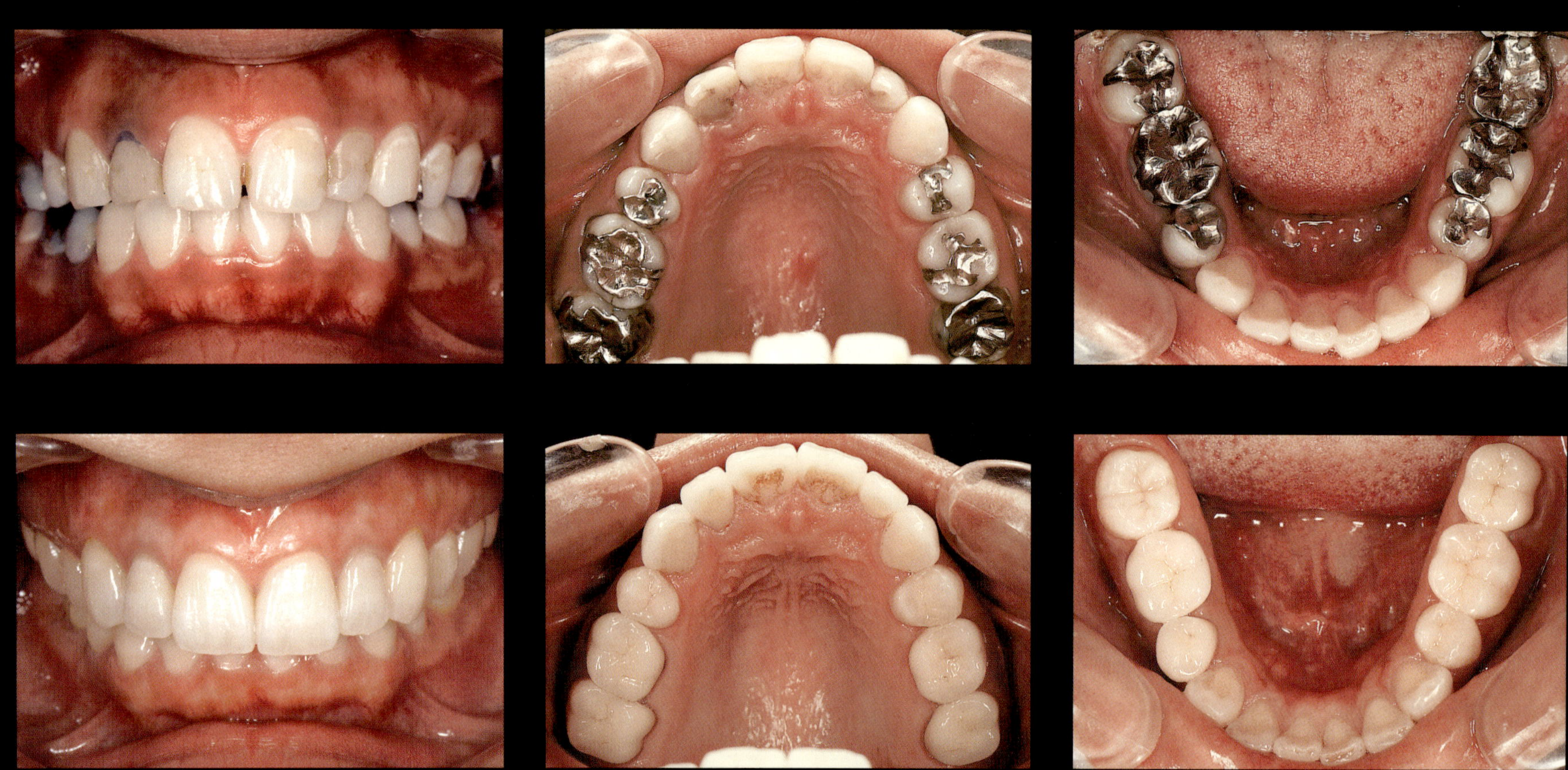

13, 11–23 porcelain veneers, 15, 25–26, 35–36 45–46 porcelain inlays and onlays, 17–16, 12, 27, 37, 46 Procera crowns

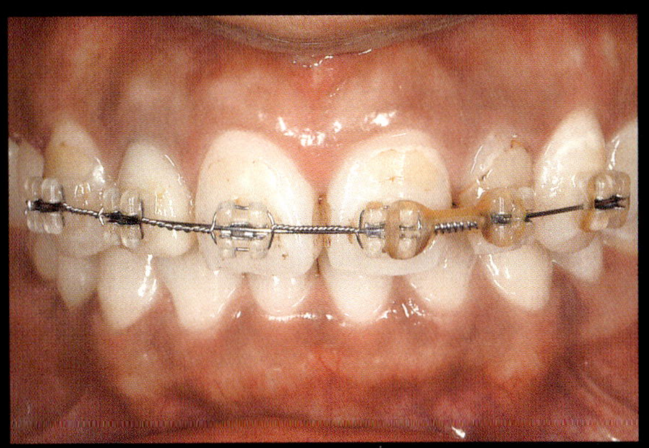

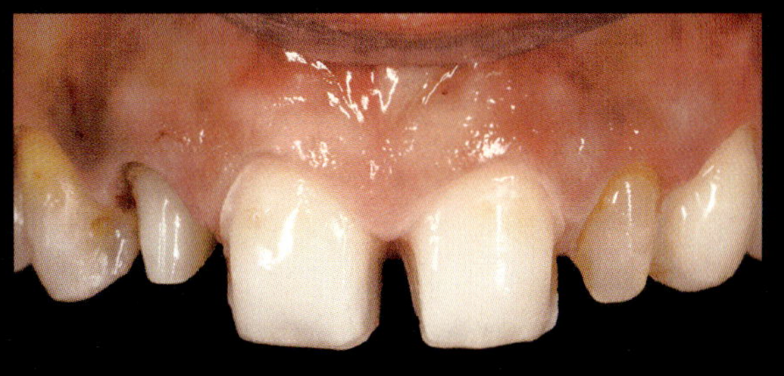

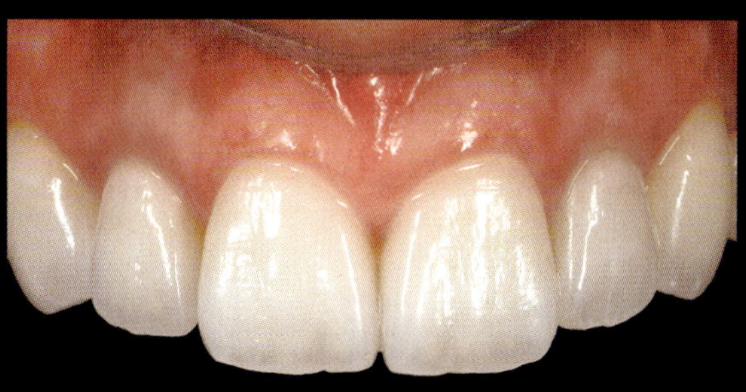

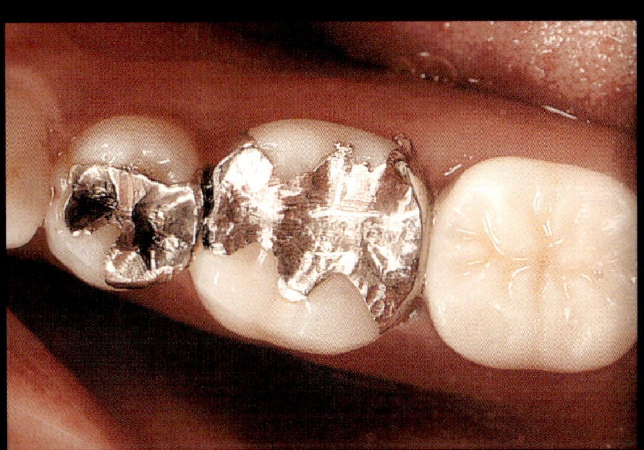

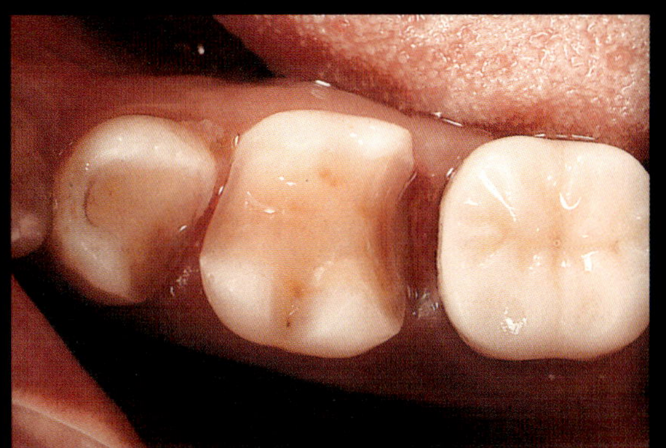

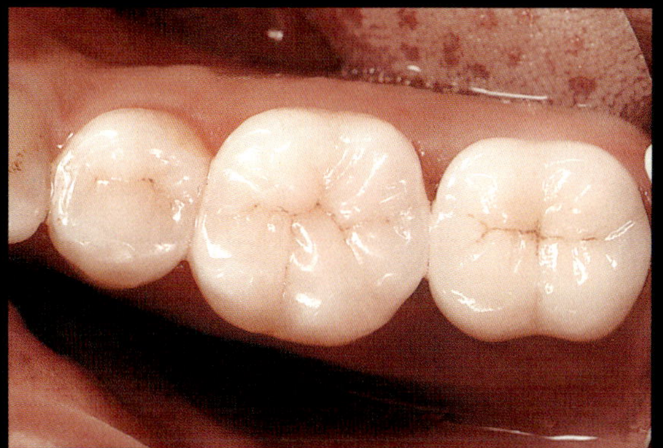

New restorations were made after the patient had completed orthodontic treatment with subsequent plastic surgical treatment and elimination of the color changes in the soft tissue.

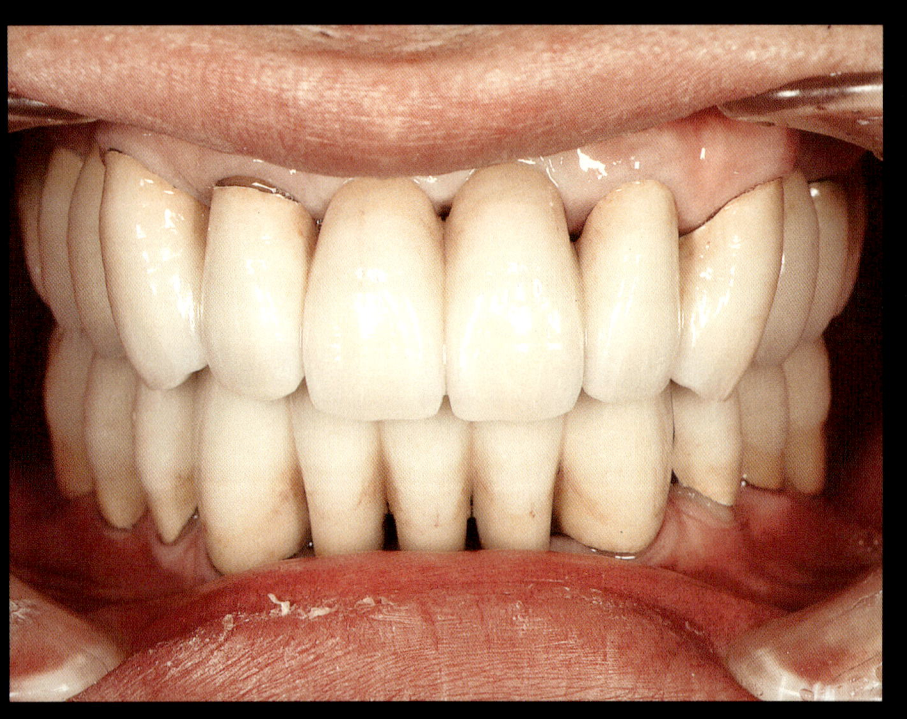
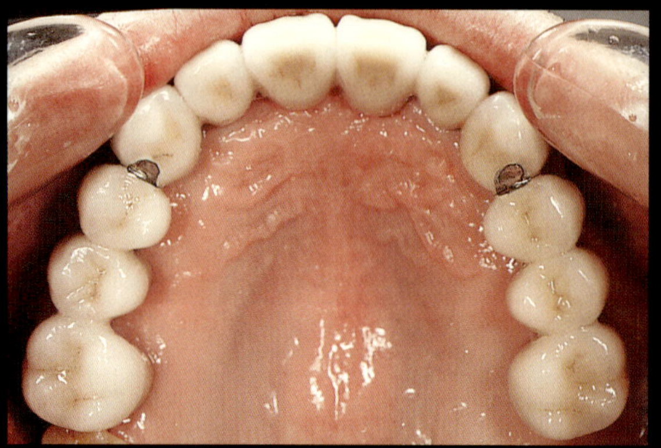
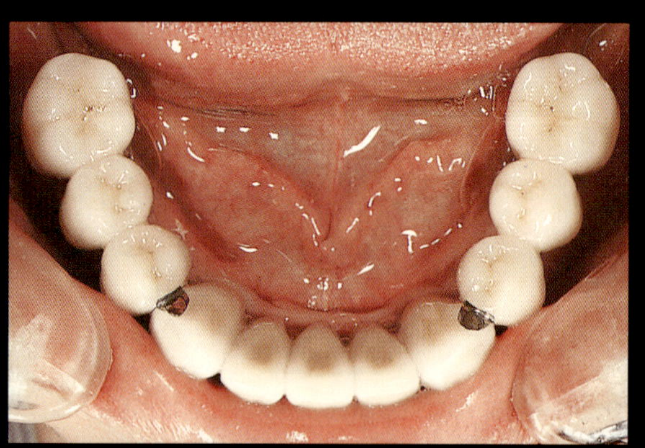

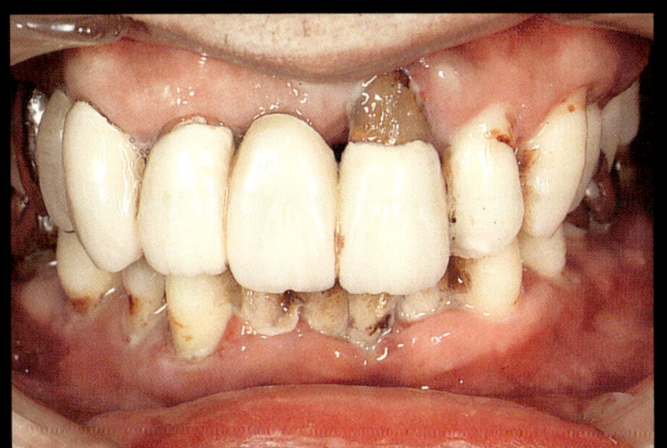
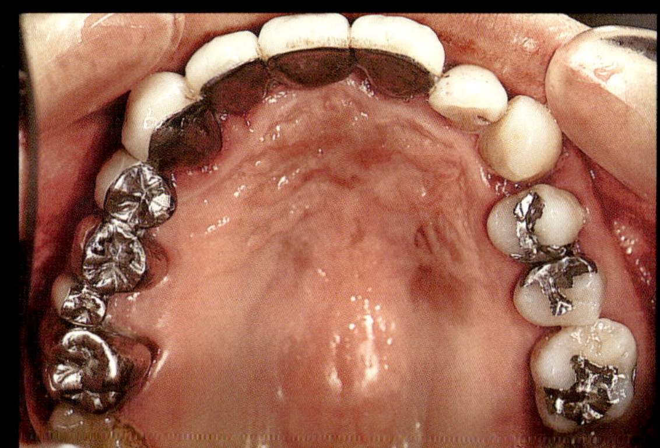
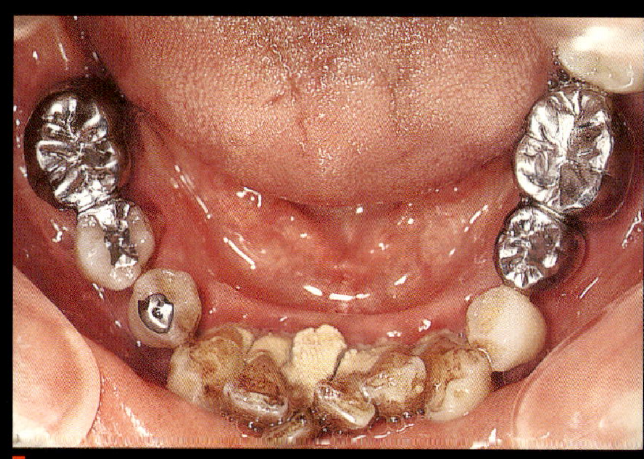
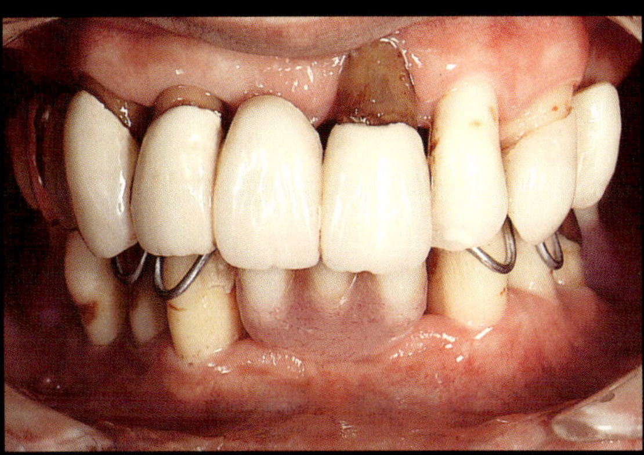

Initial treatment

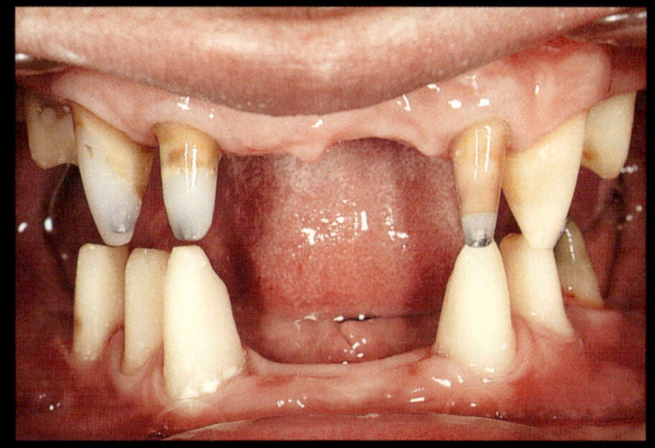

After surgery

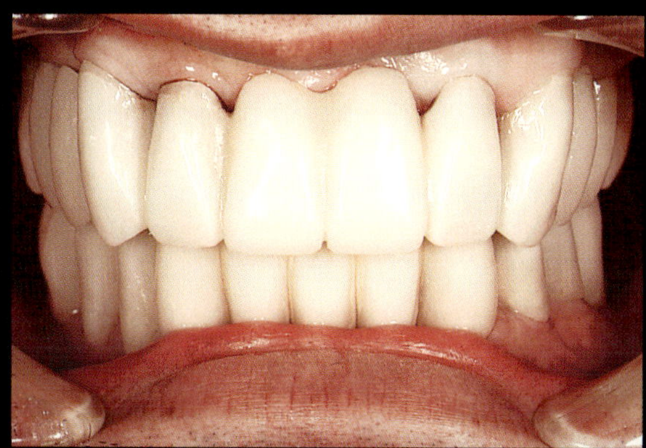

Temporary restoration

Periodontal prostheses

Periodontal prostheses are increasingly losing their significance due to the numerous advances made in restorative implantology. Many patients, however, do not want to have foreign bodies (implants) in their mouths, but would rather keep their own teeth for as long as possible.

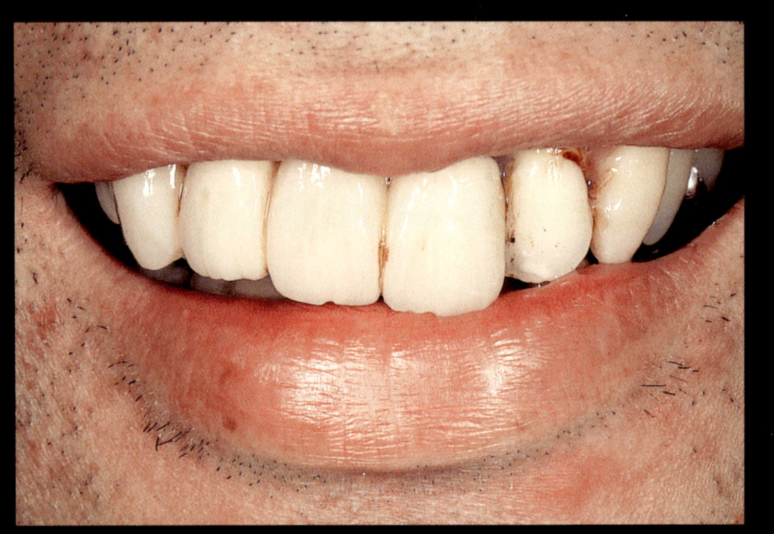

2001

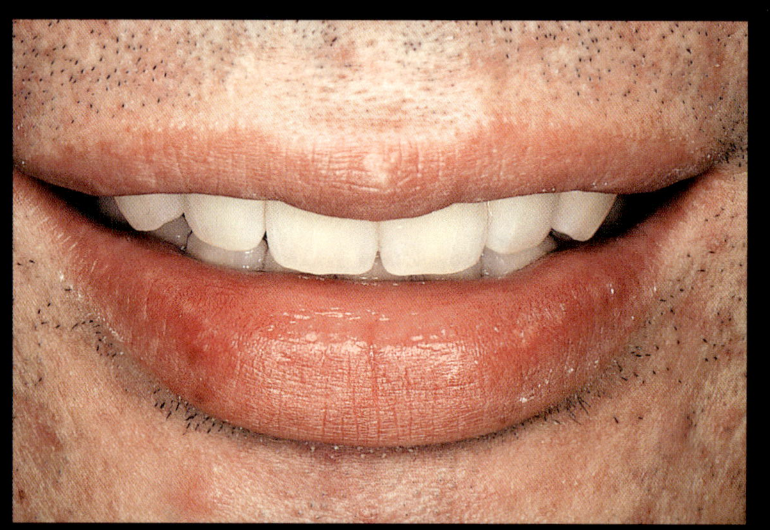

2007

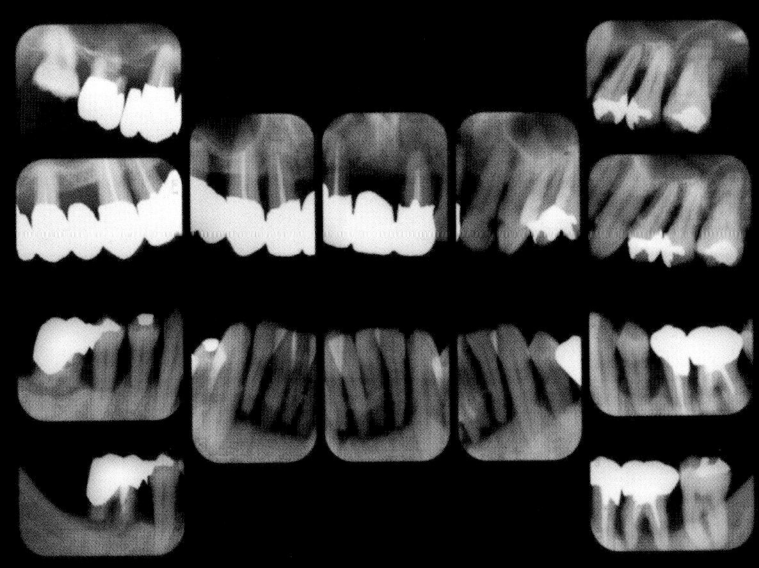

2001

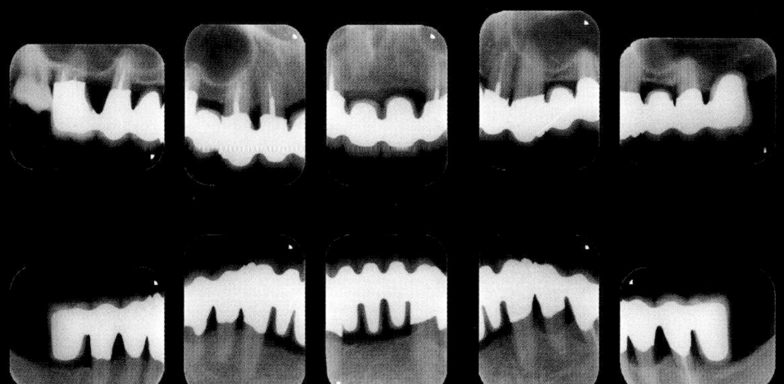

2007

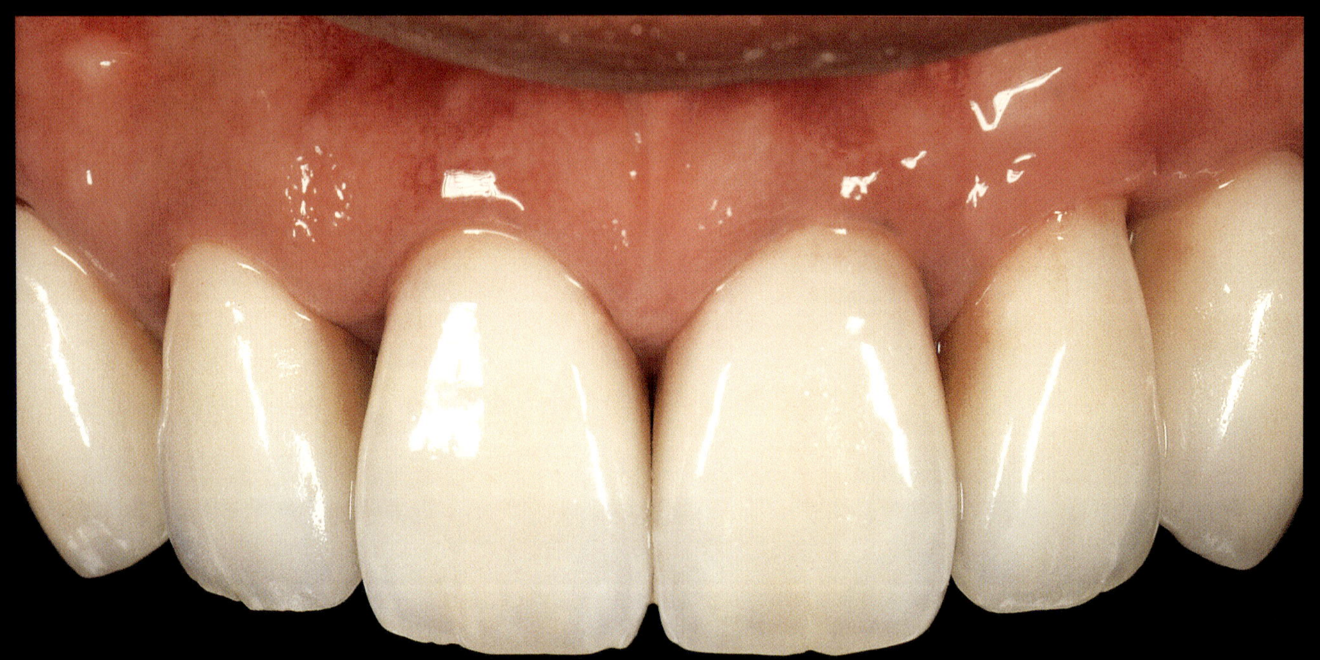

Implants

Plastic periodontal surgery and oral surgery techniques developed in recent years now make it possible to achieve implantological restoration results that are comparable to those of natural tooth restorations.

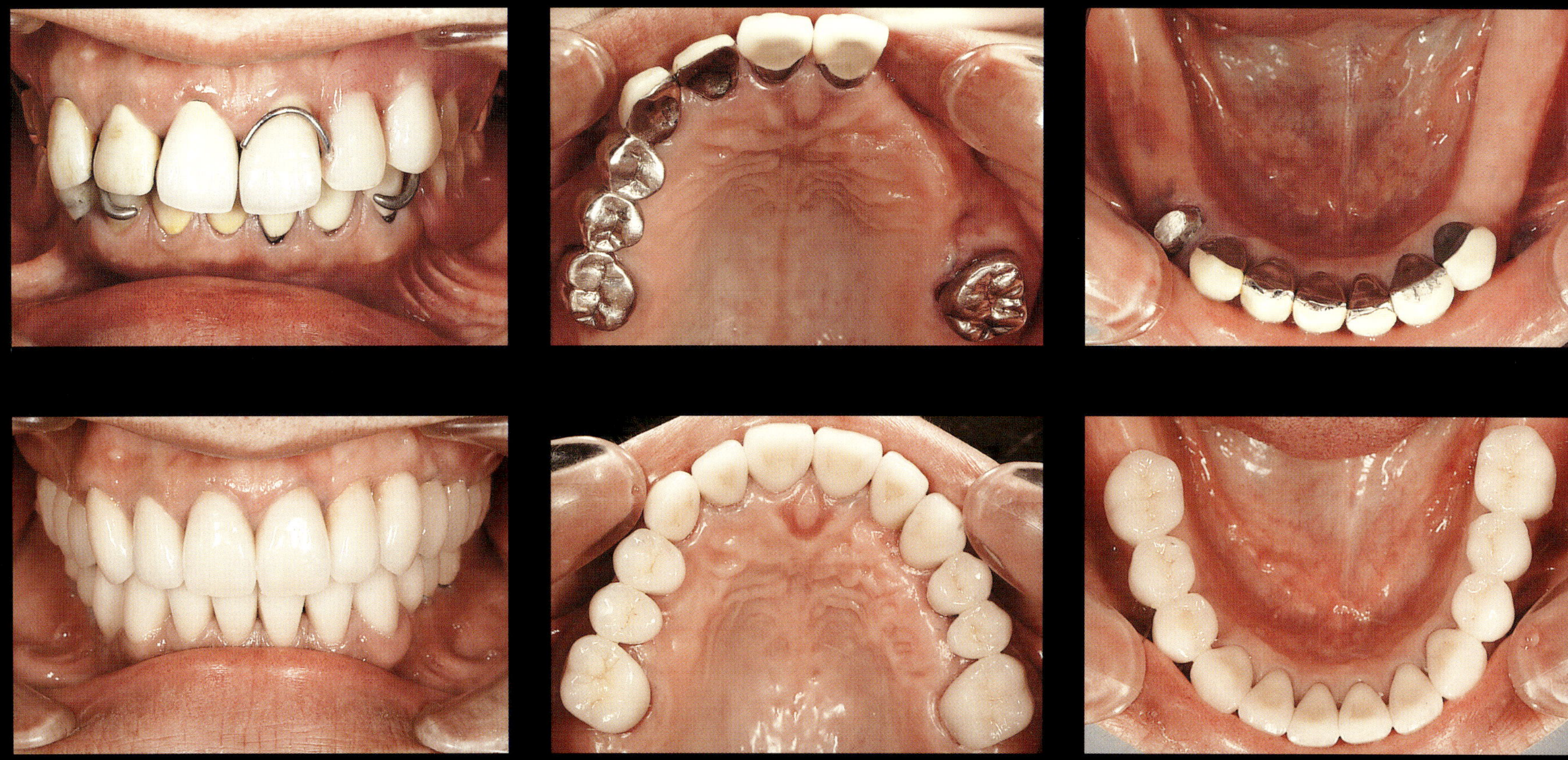

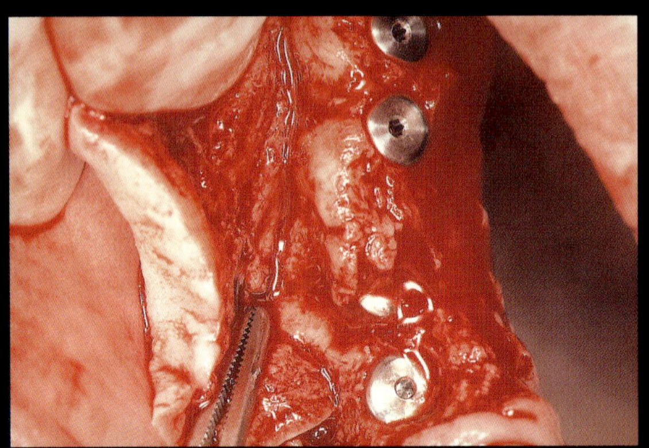

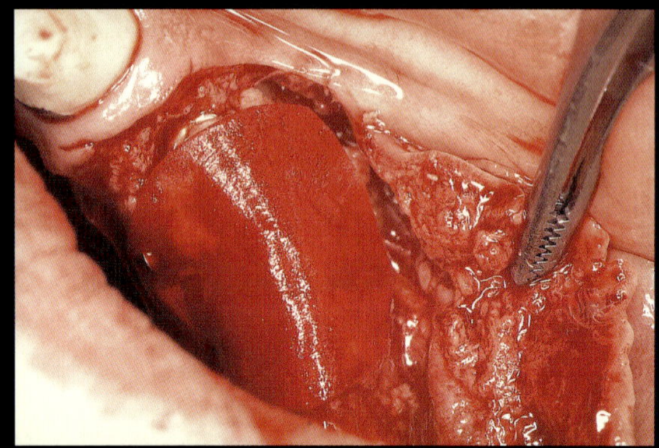

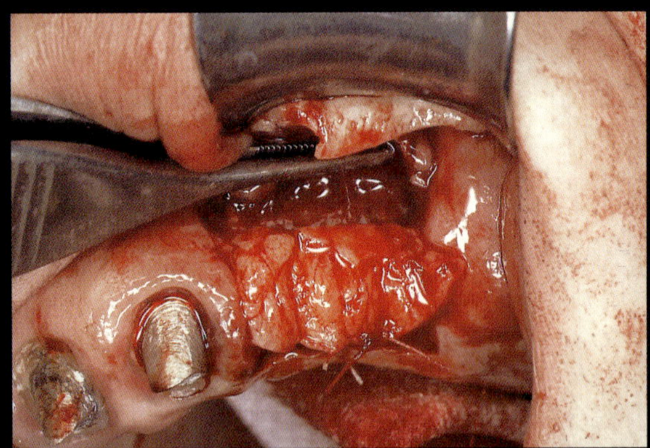

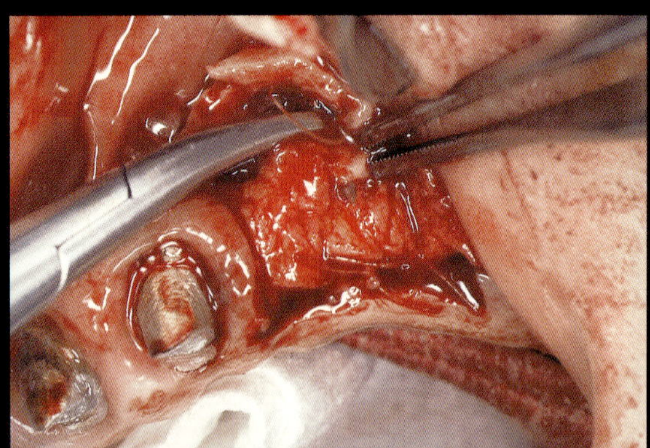

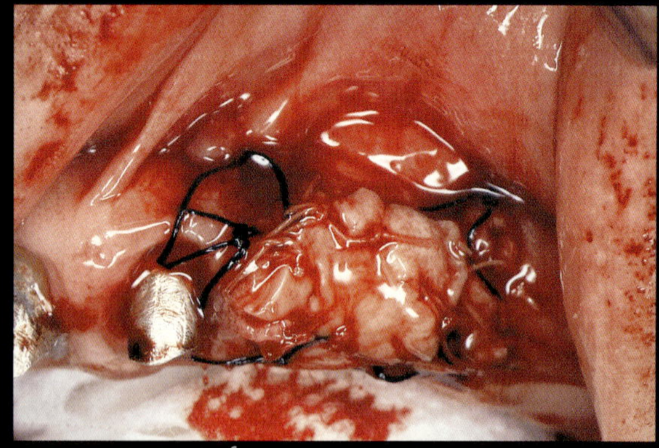

With implant insertion, controlled bone regeneration is initiated with autologous bone graft material in order to build up the hard tissue. Connective tissue inlay and onlay grafts were used to increase keratinized gingiva for restoration of esthetics.

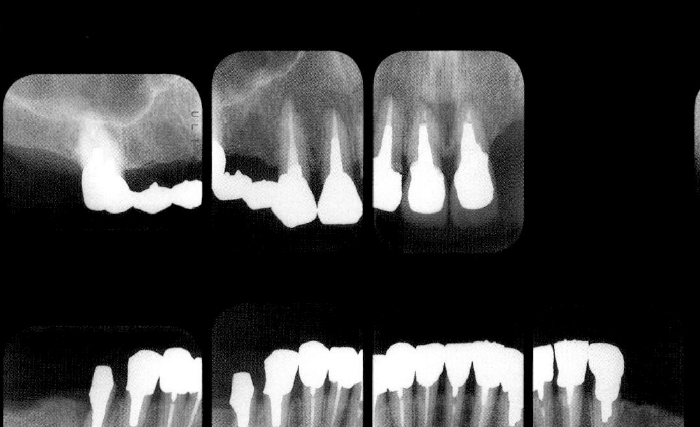

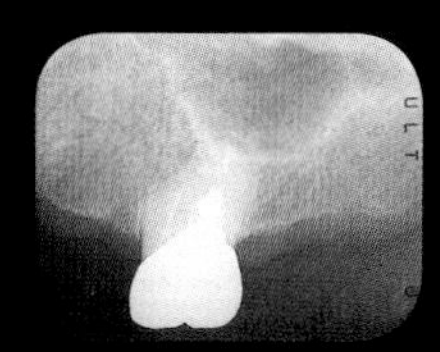

2002

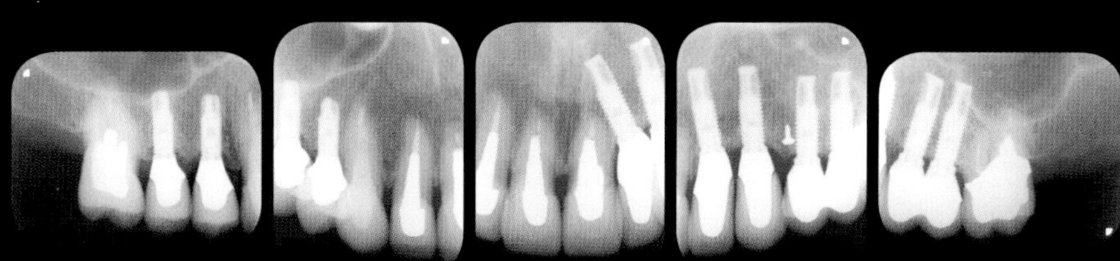

2007

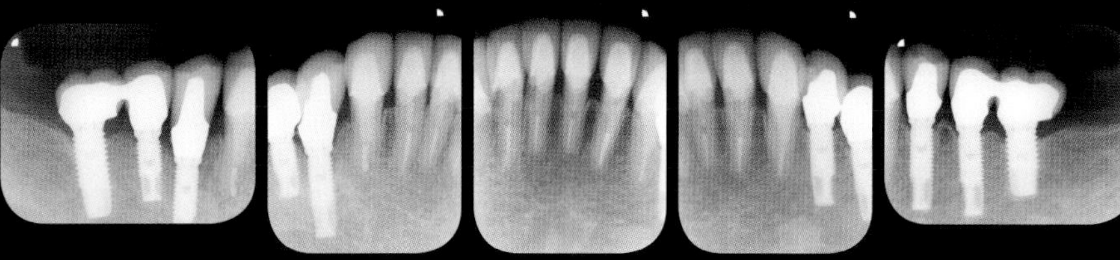

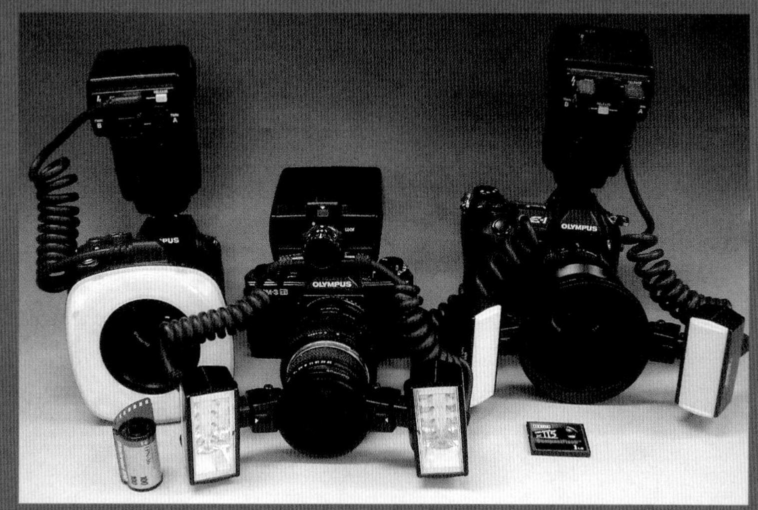

Photographic equipment and materials

OLYMPUS E-500
50 mm f2.0 MACRO

OM-3
80 mm f4.0 MACRO
Film: Kodak EPN 100

E-1
50 mm f2.0 MACRO

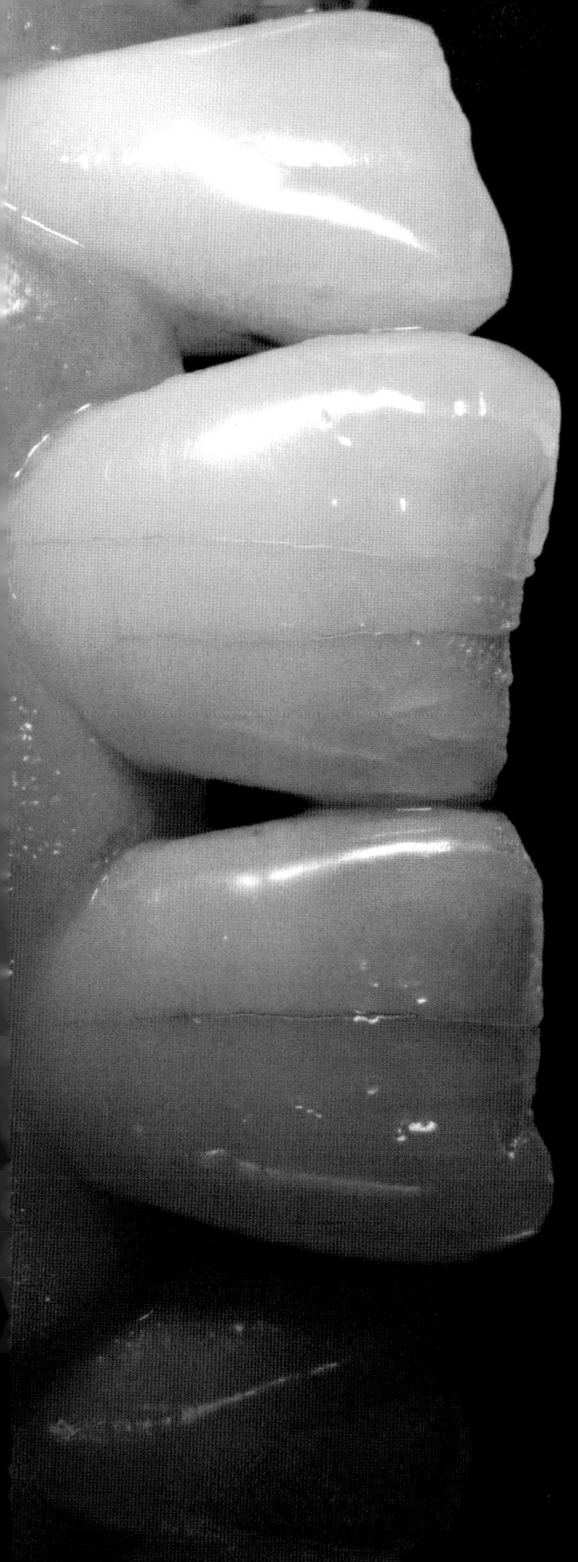

10 Intact teeth

Healthy teeth vary in appearance, color, shape, surface structure and other characteristics. The diversity of natural teeth serves as the model for restorative dentistry -- and for our dreams.

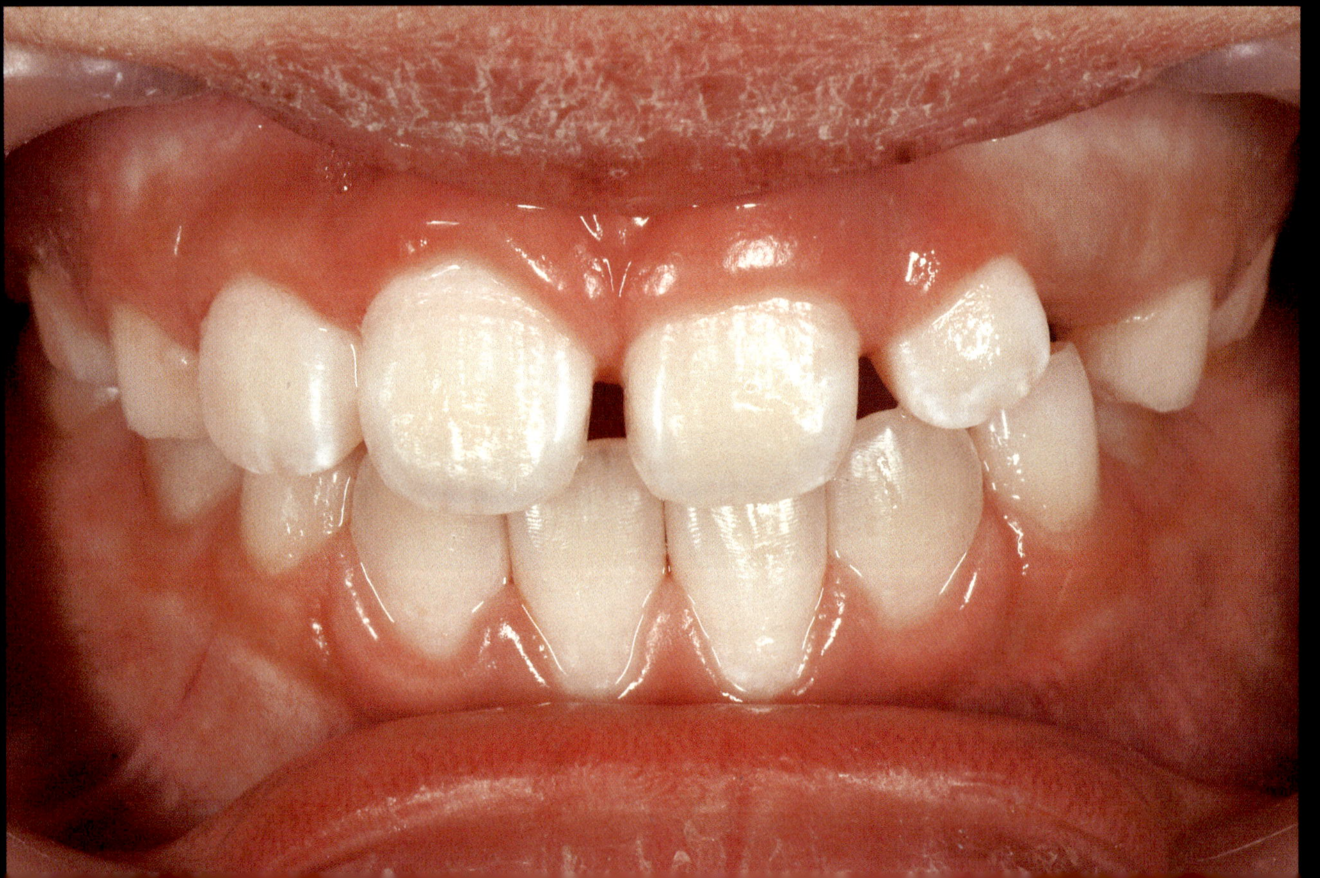

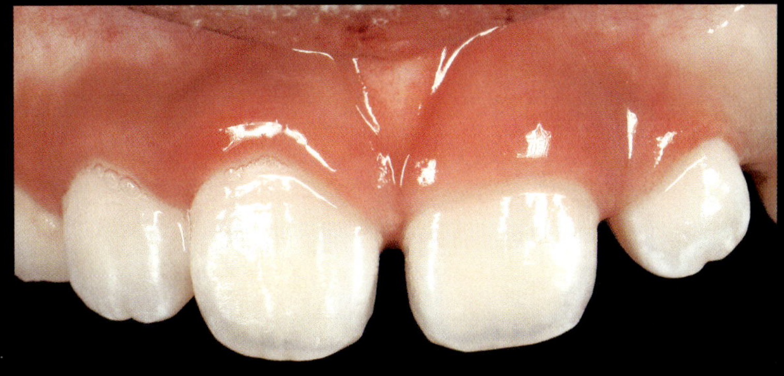

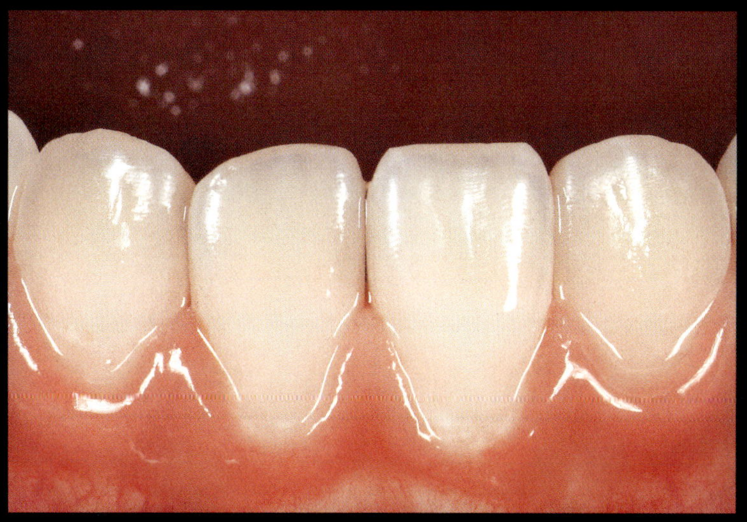

6-year-old female

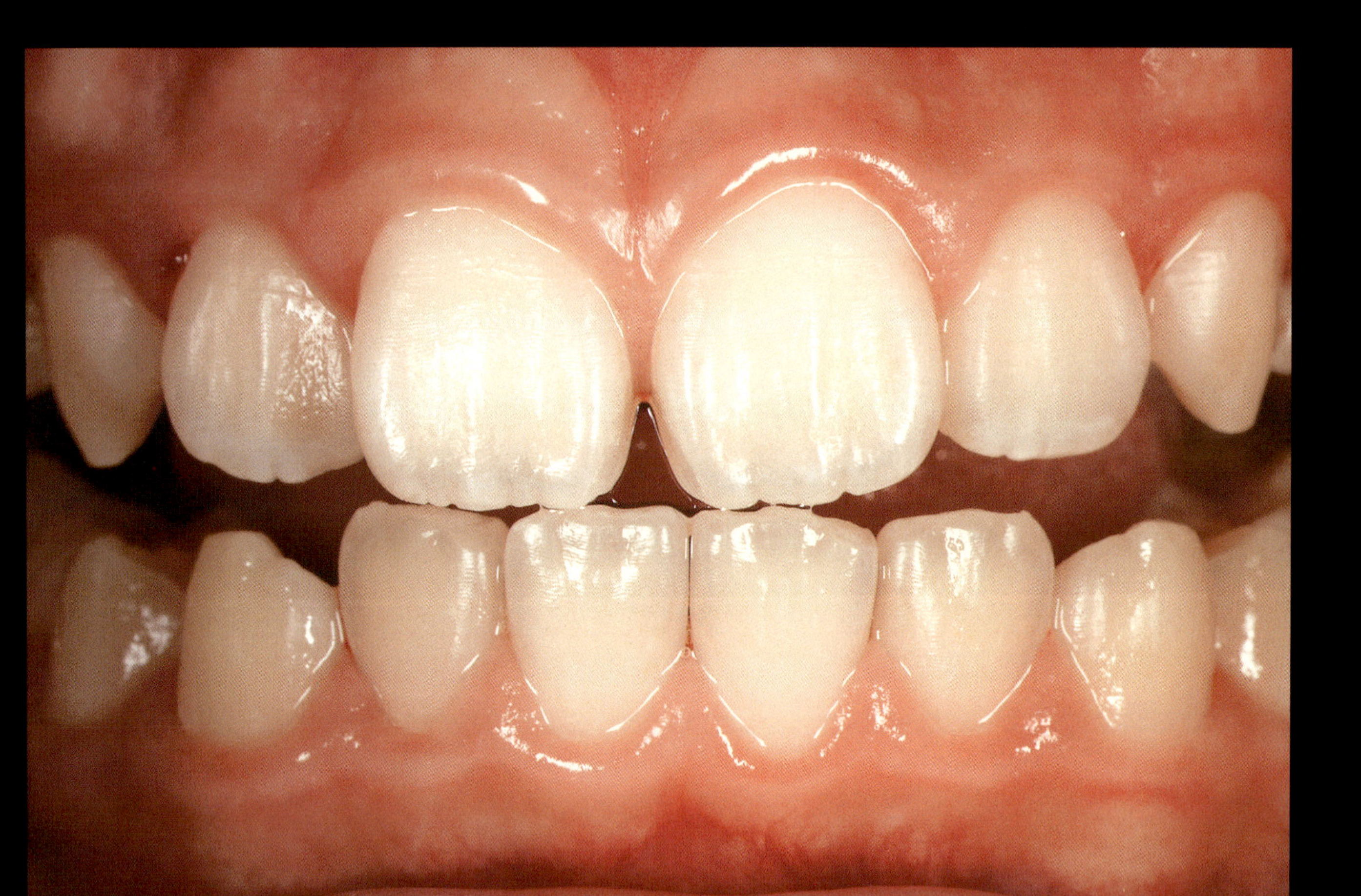

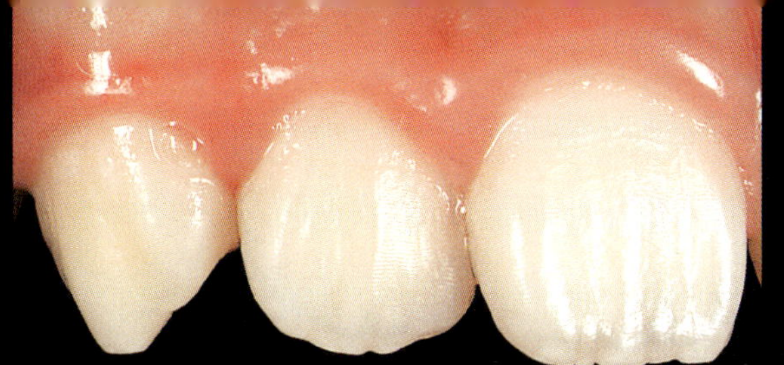
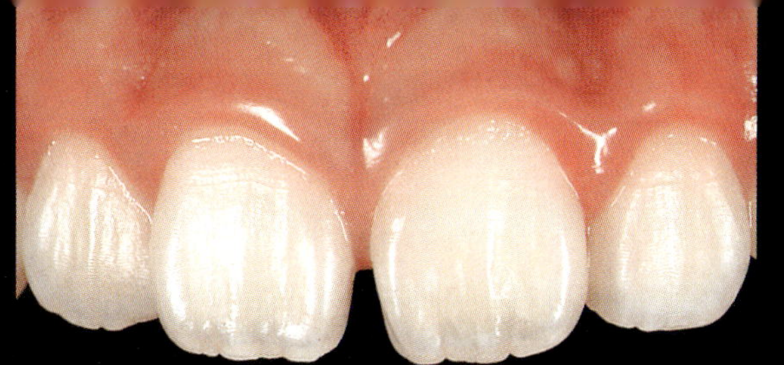
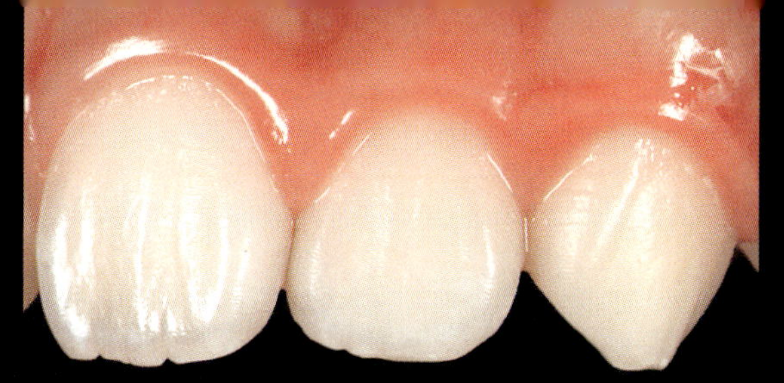
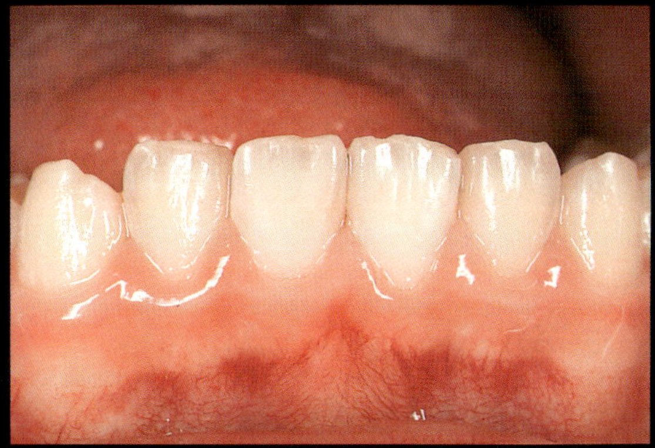
11-year-old female

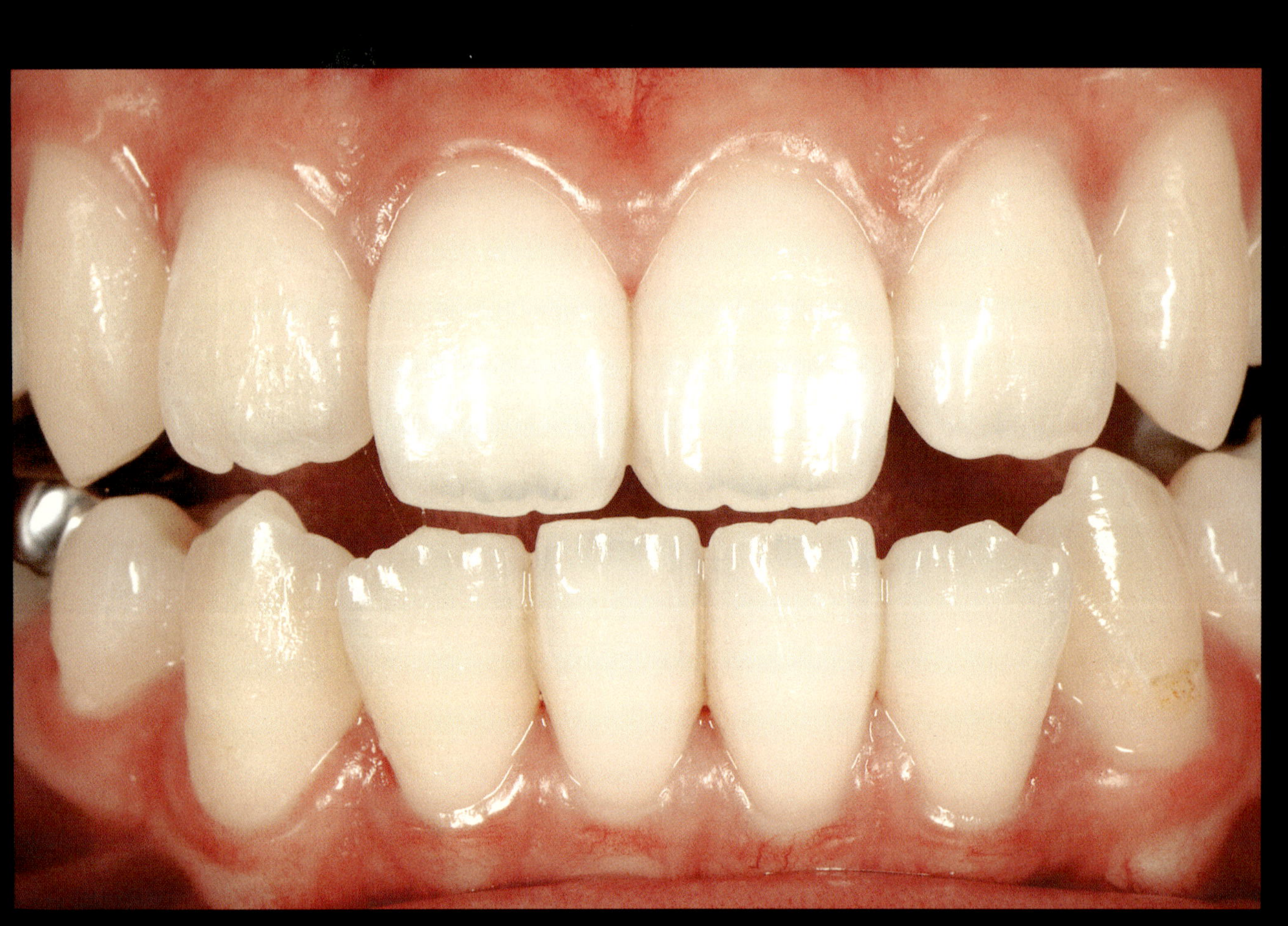

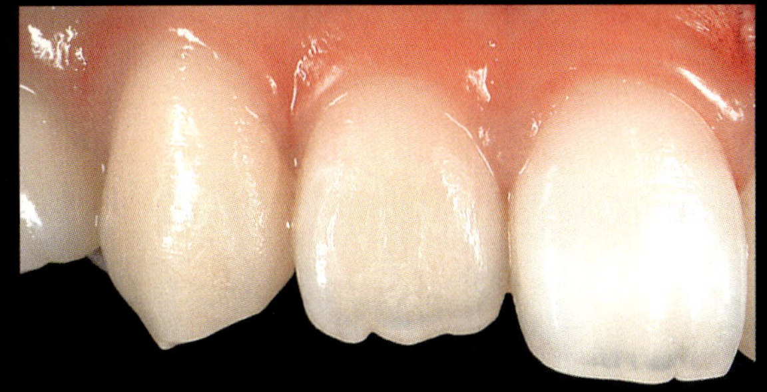

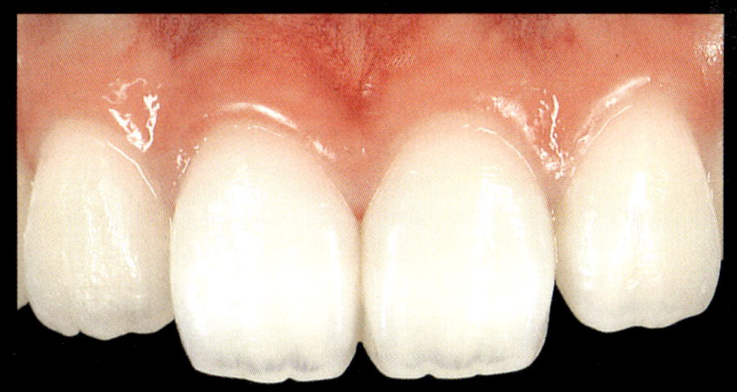

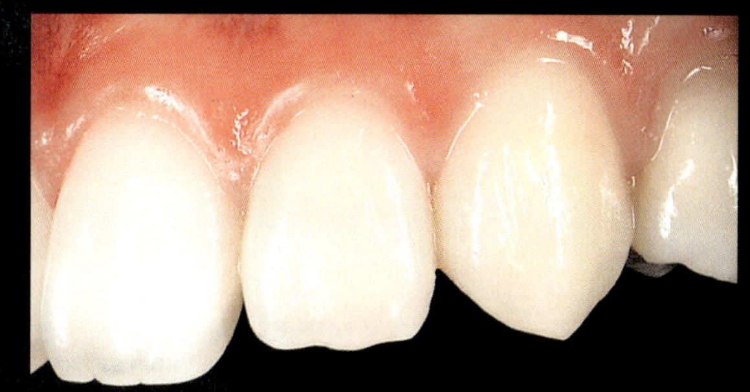

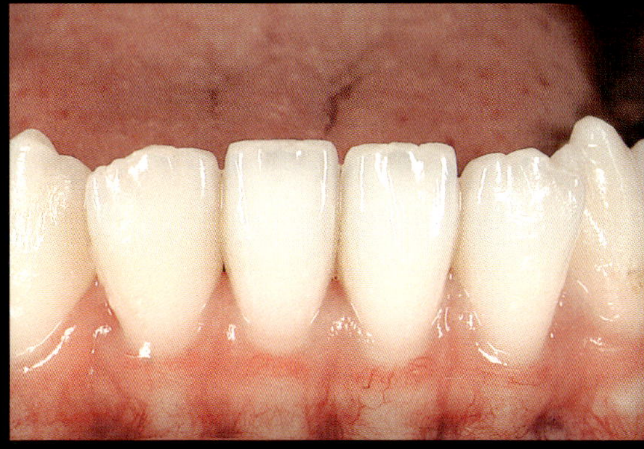

18-year-old female

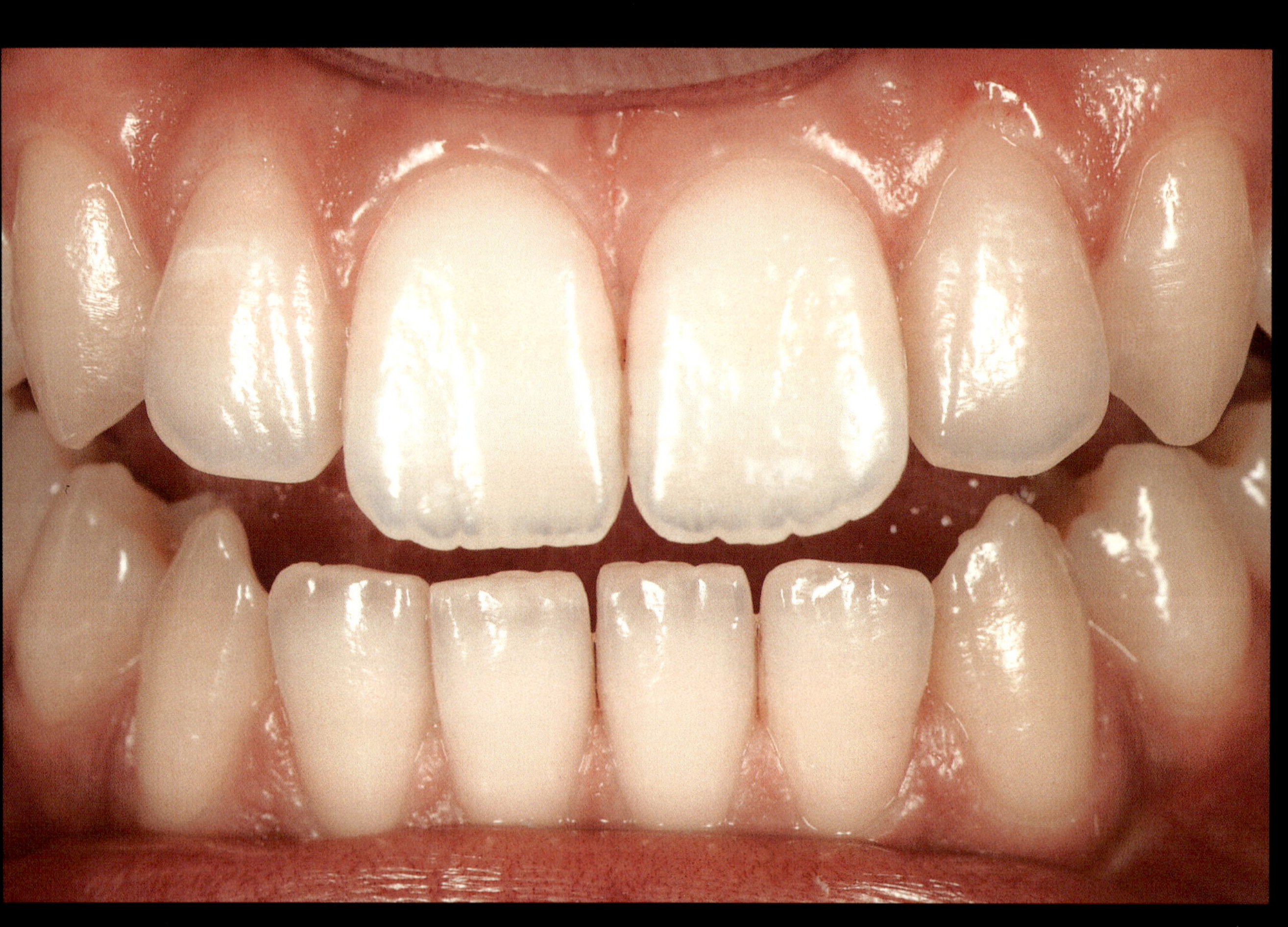

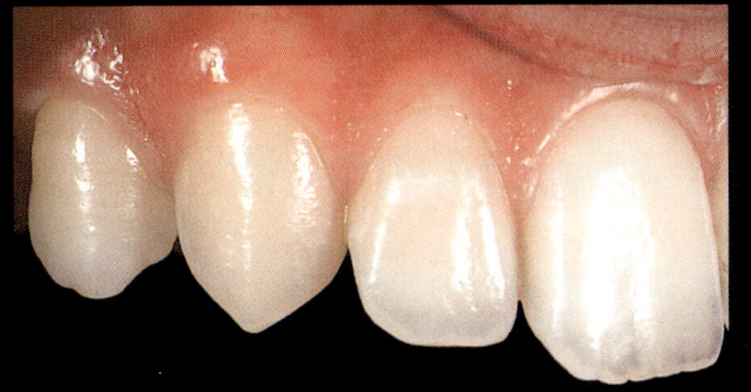
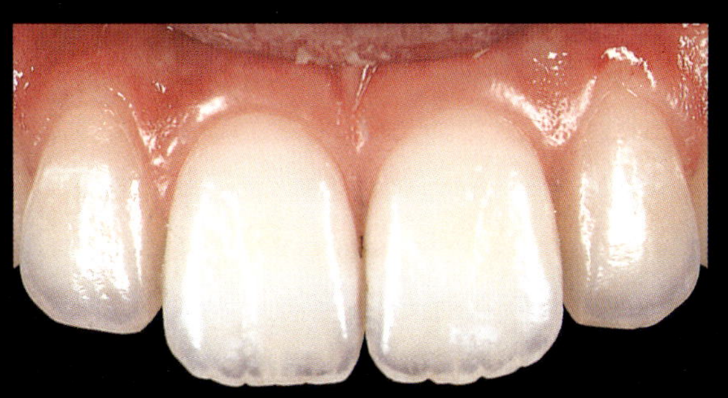
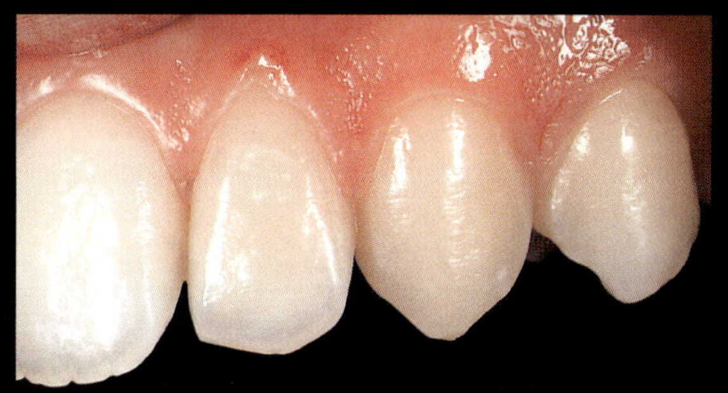
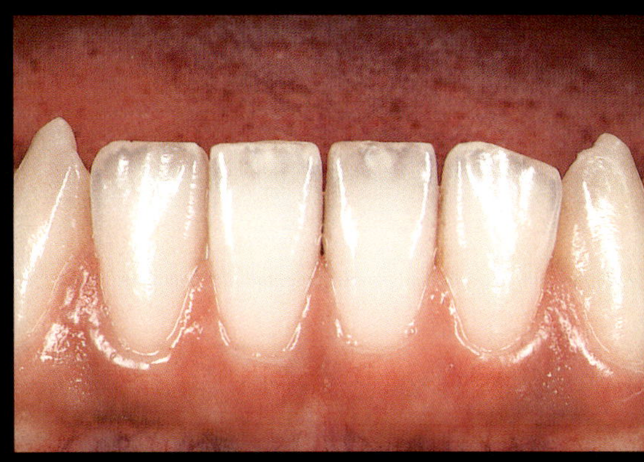

19-year-old female

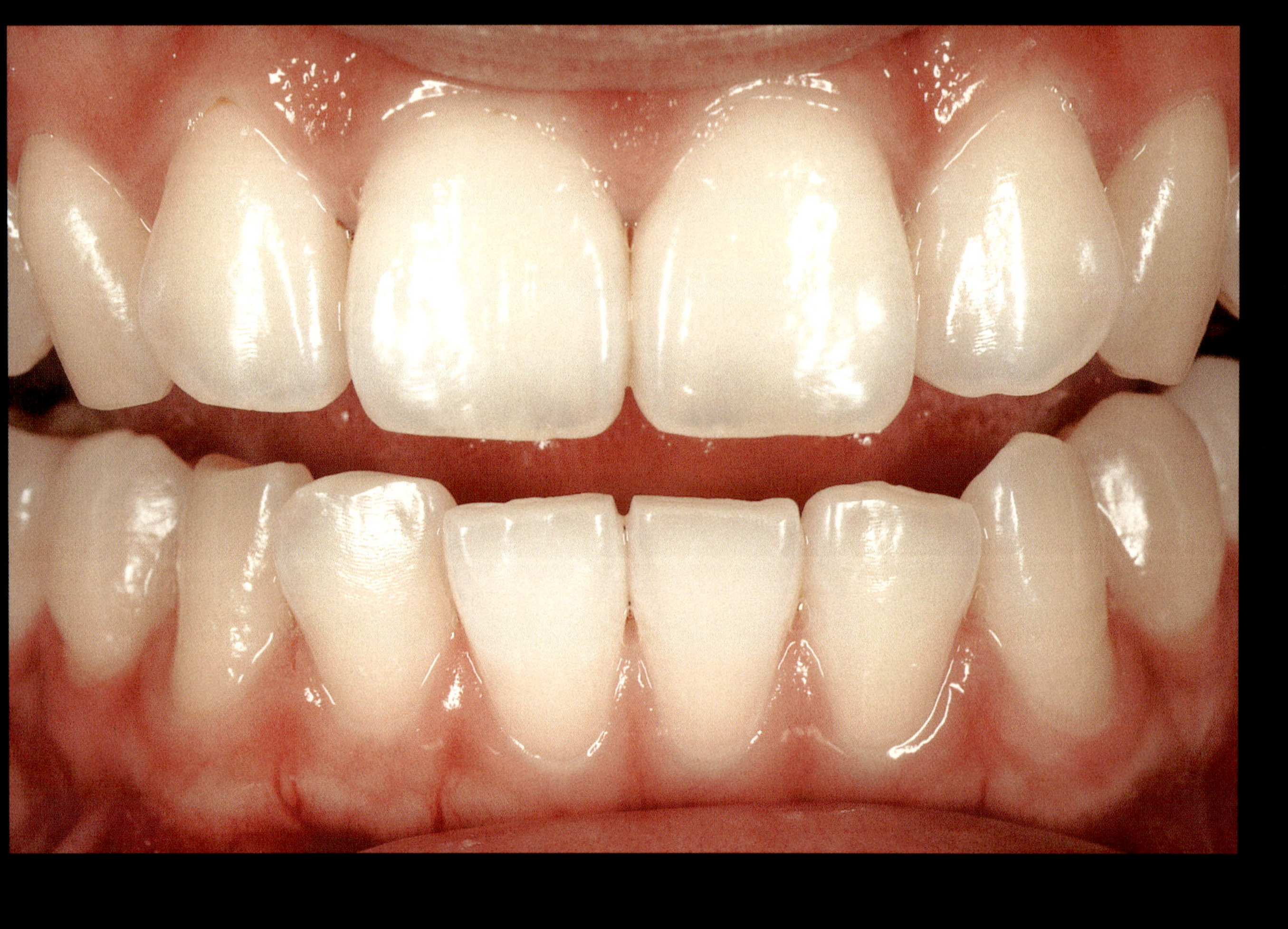

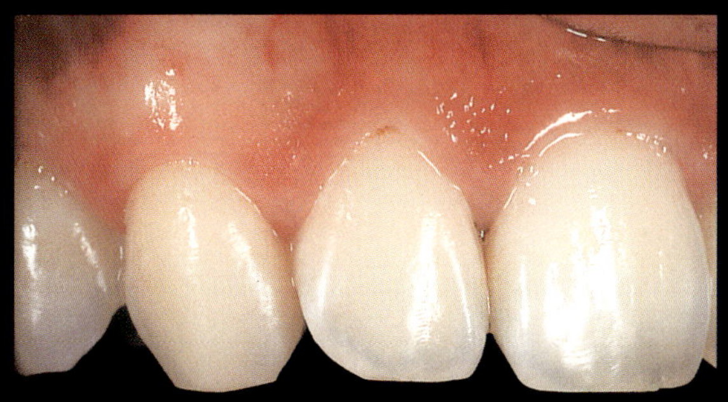

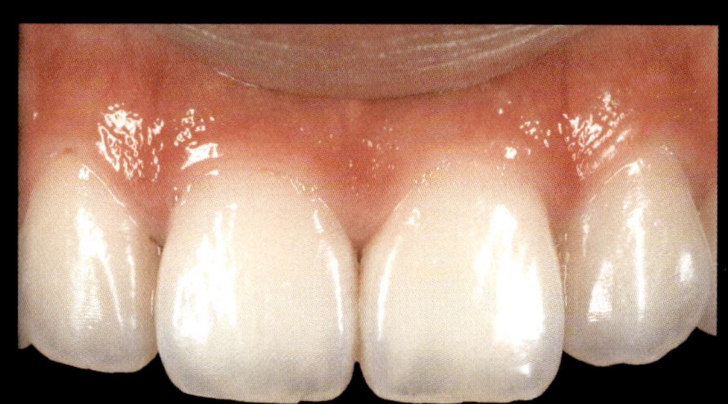

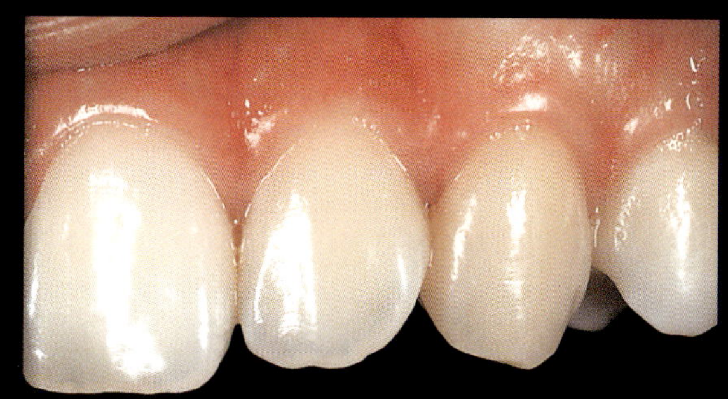

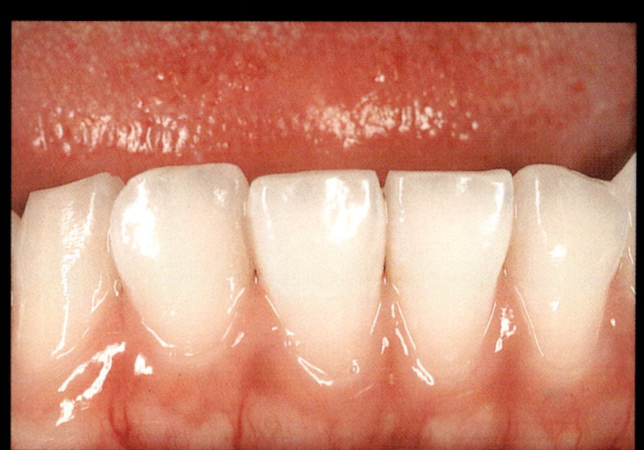

23-year-old female

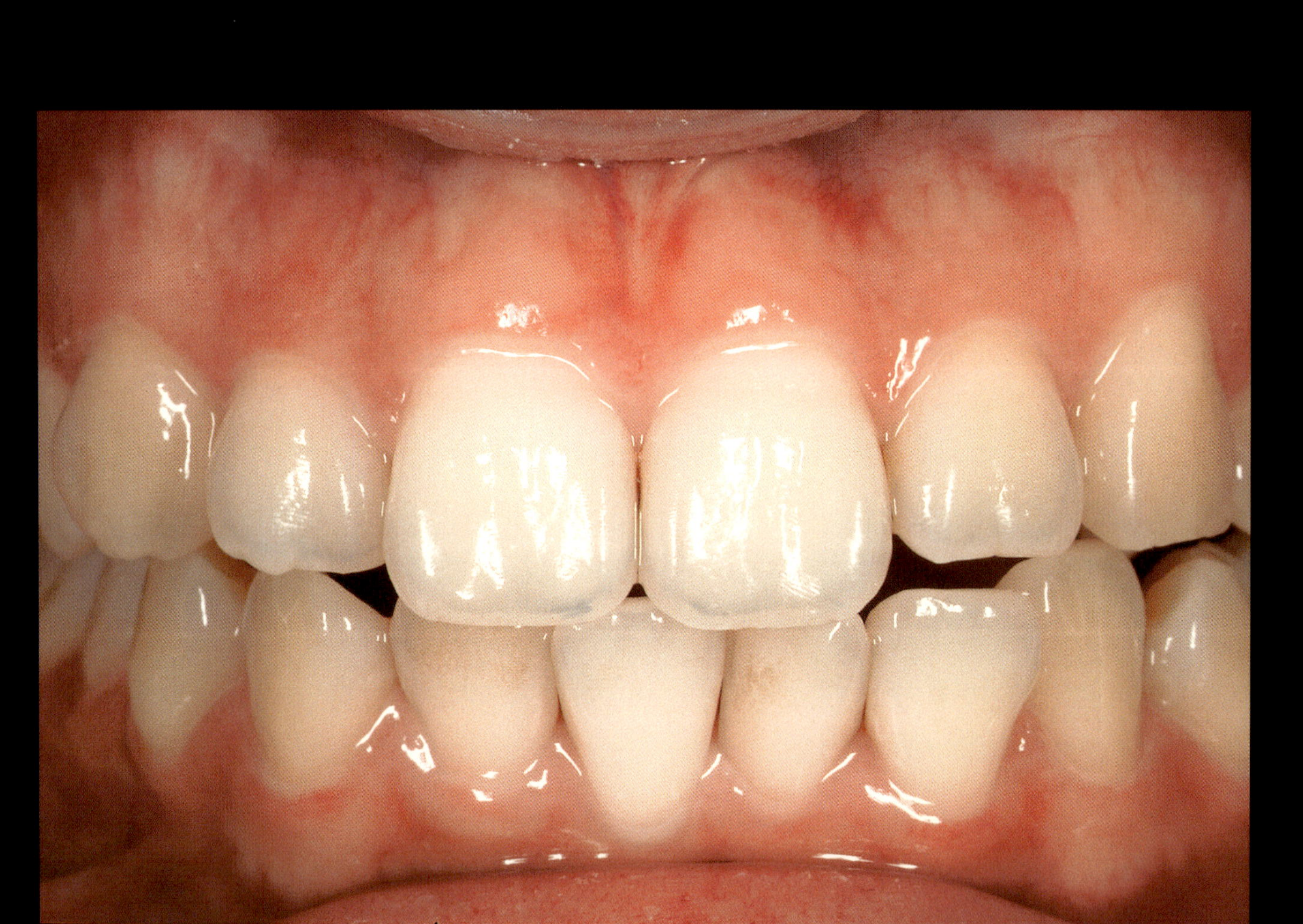

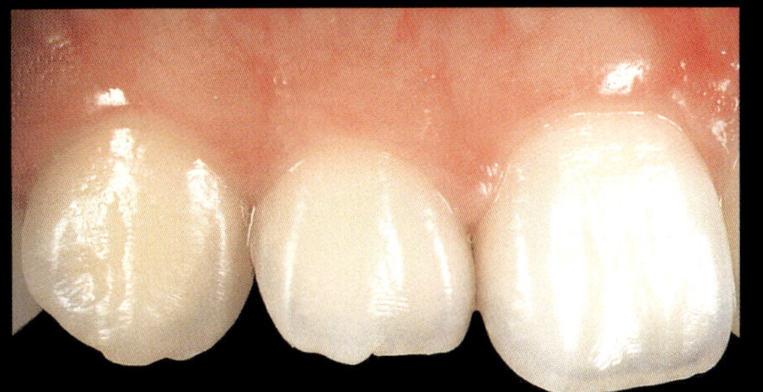

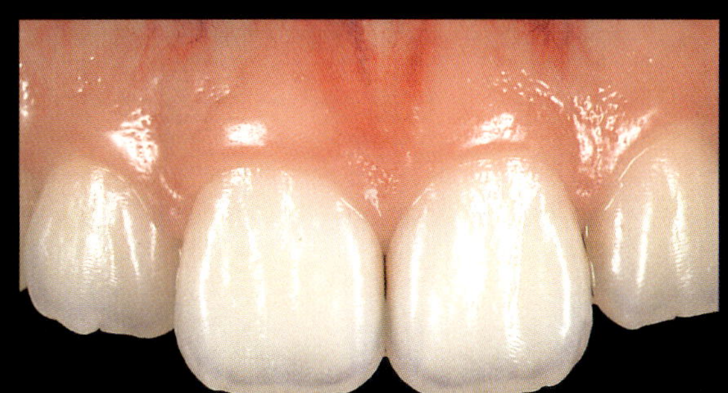

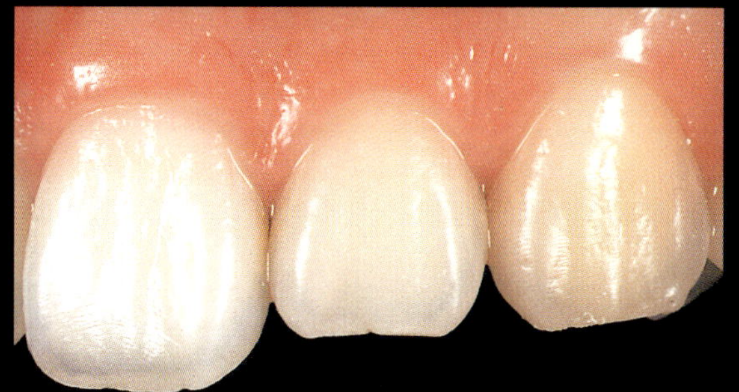

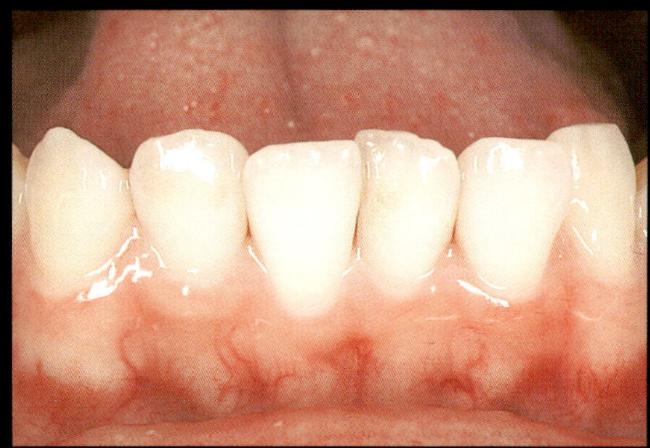

24-year-old female

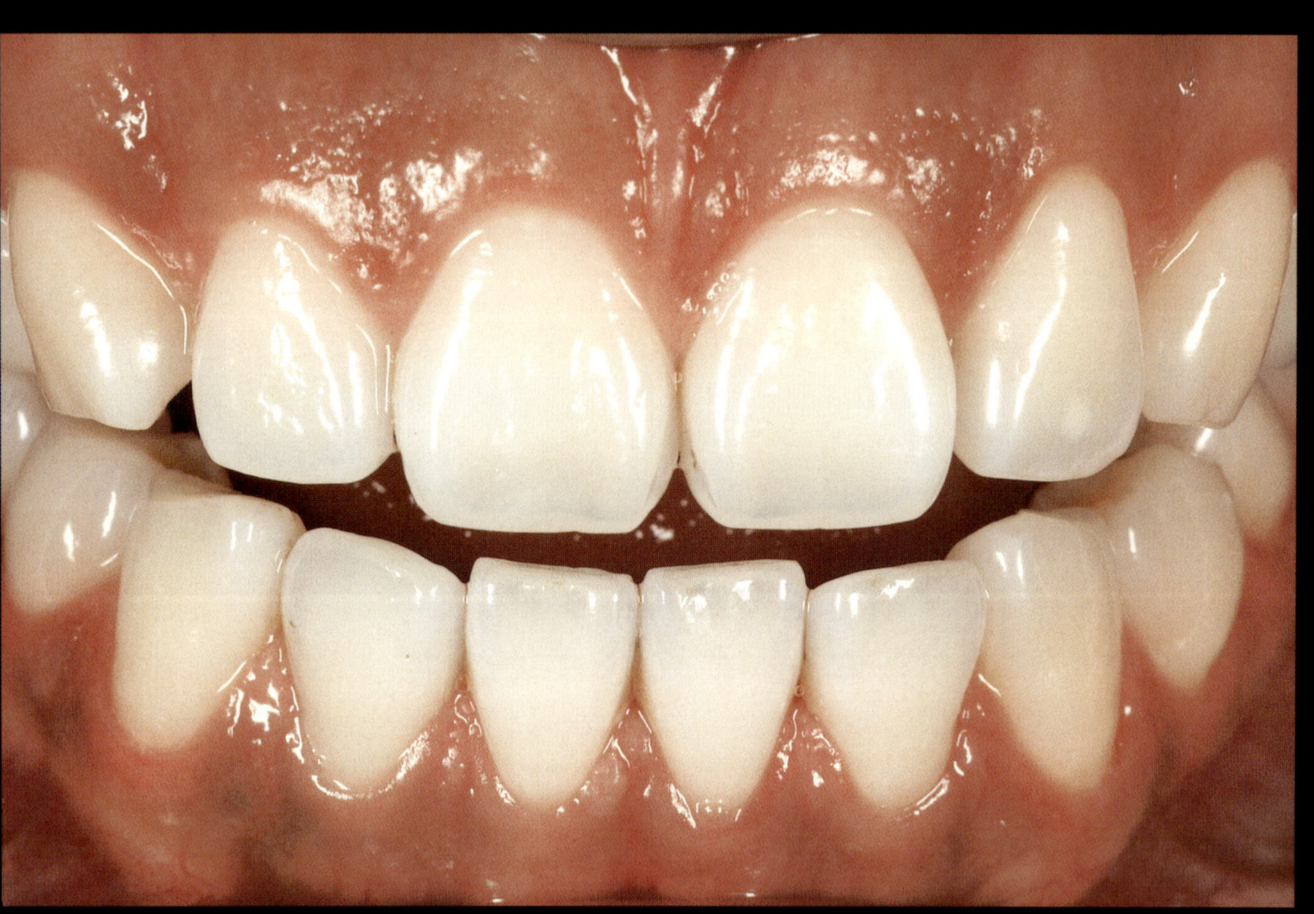

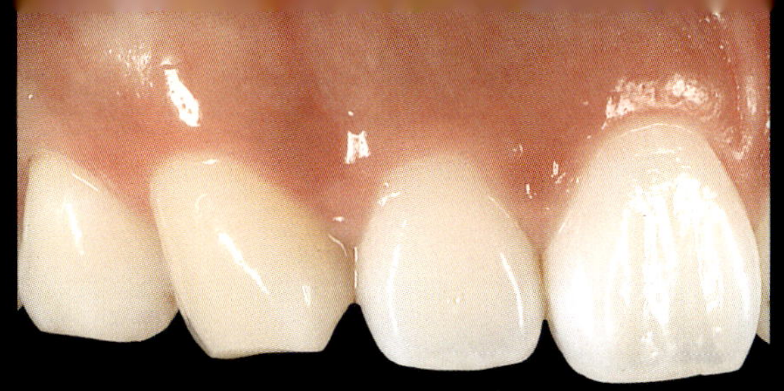

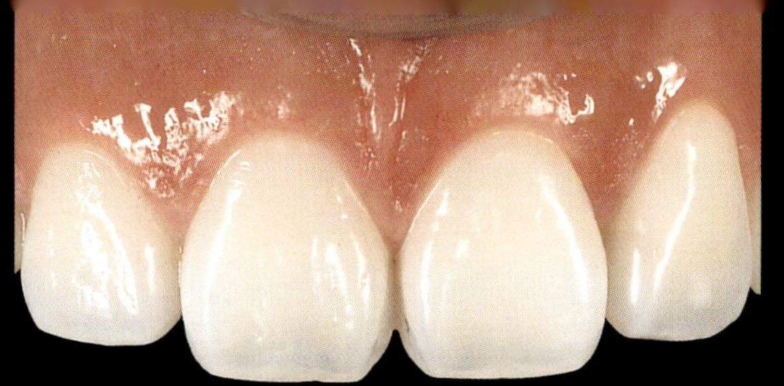

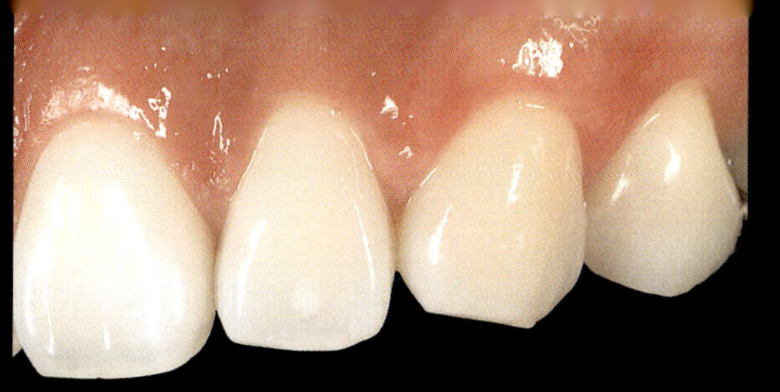

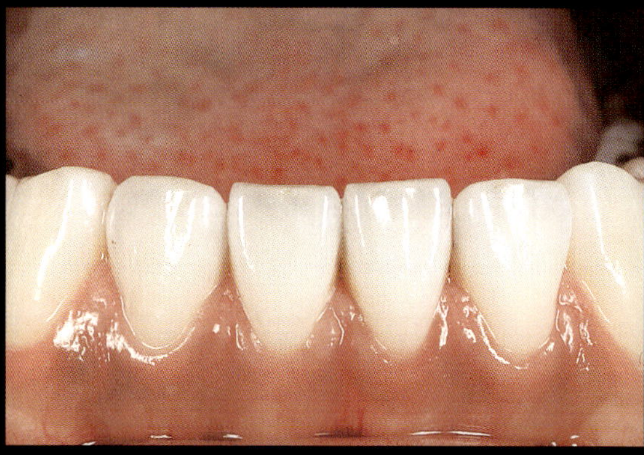

25-year-old female

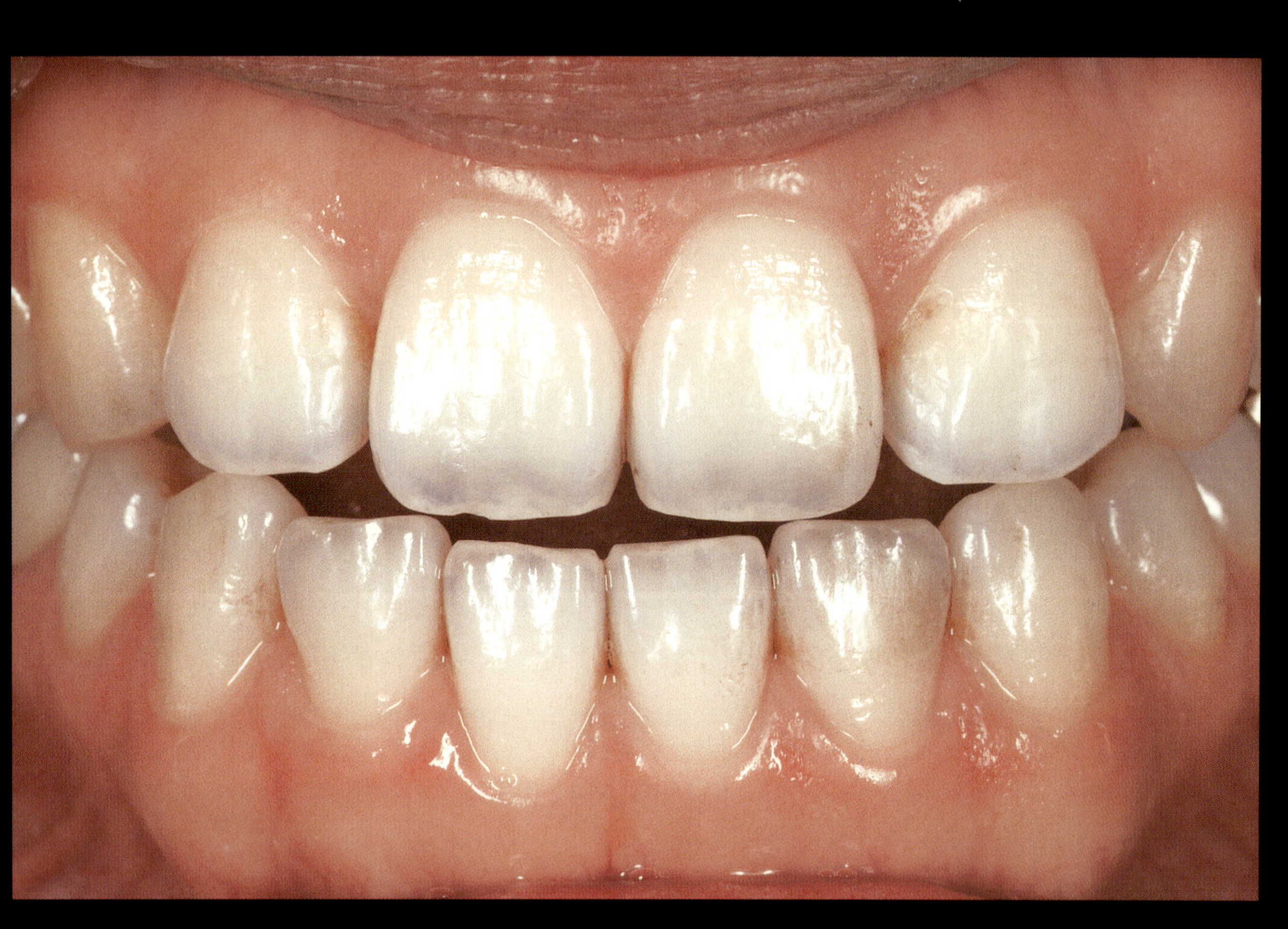

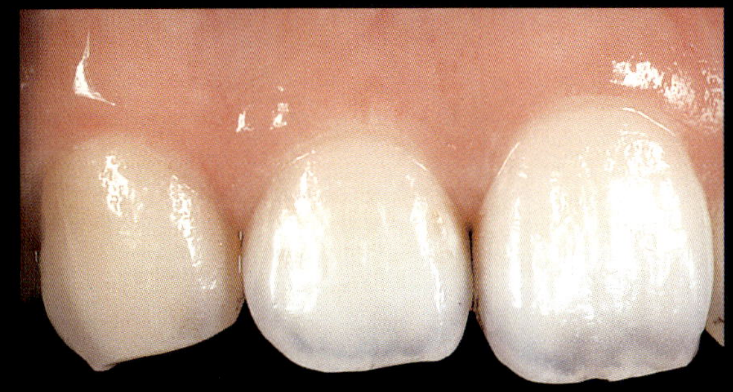

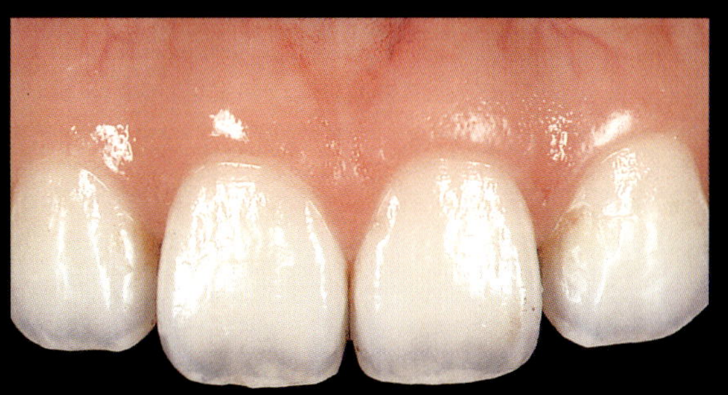

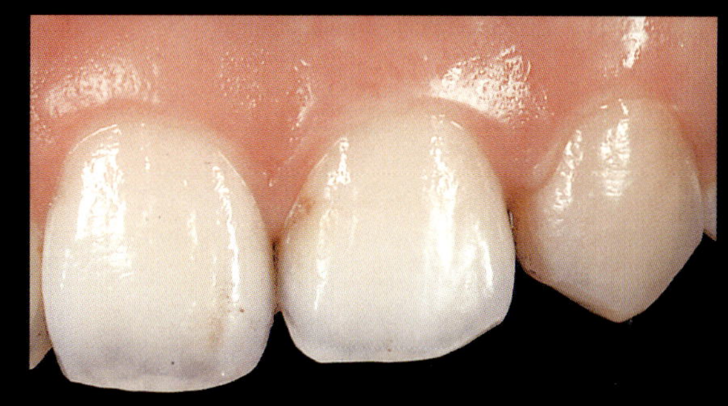

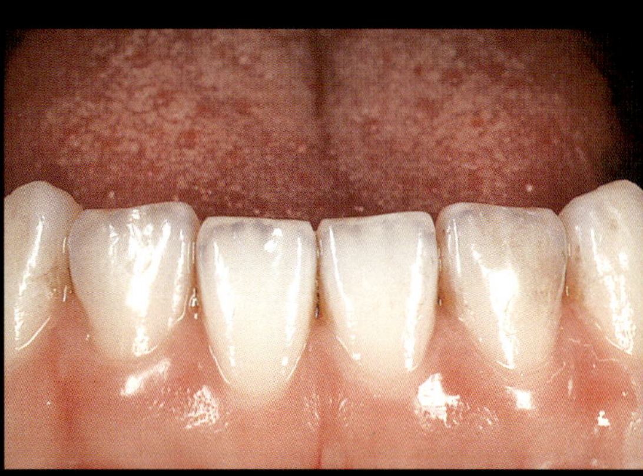

26-year-old female

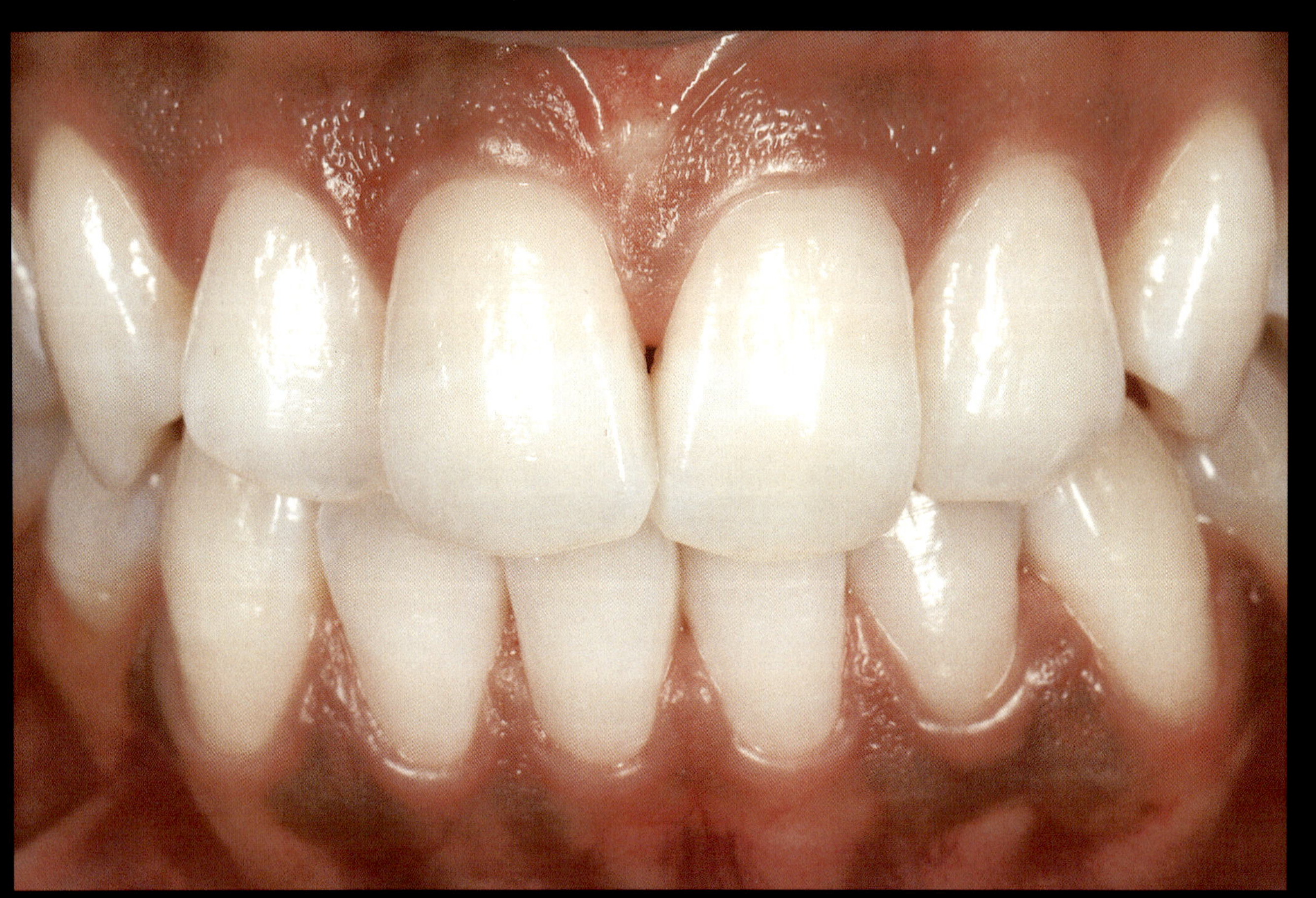

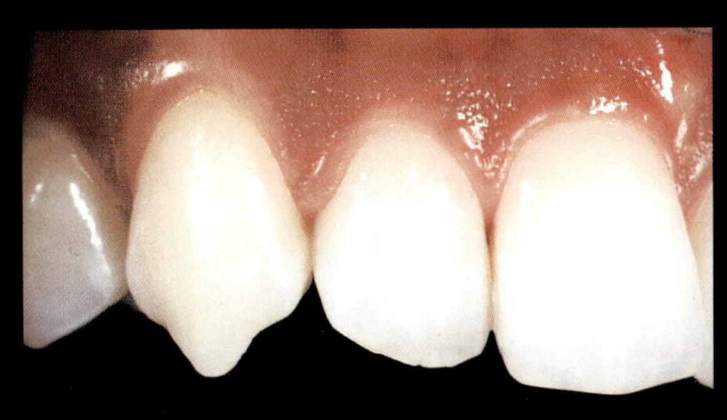

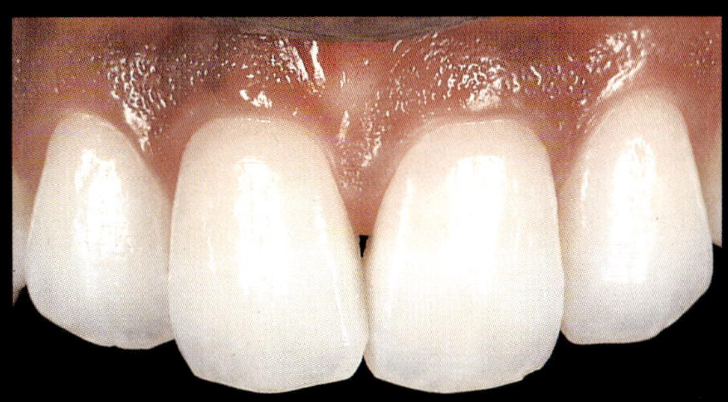

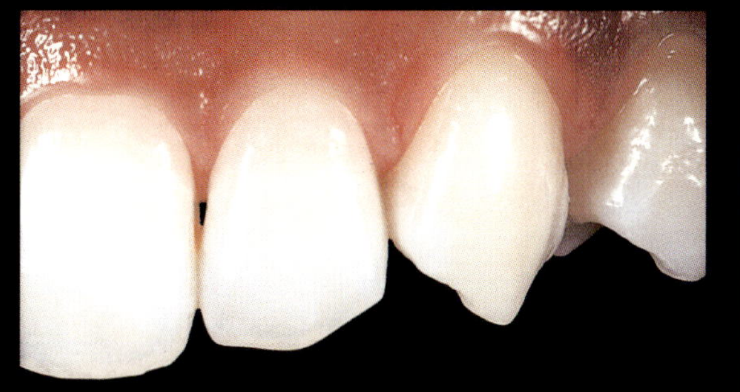

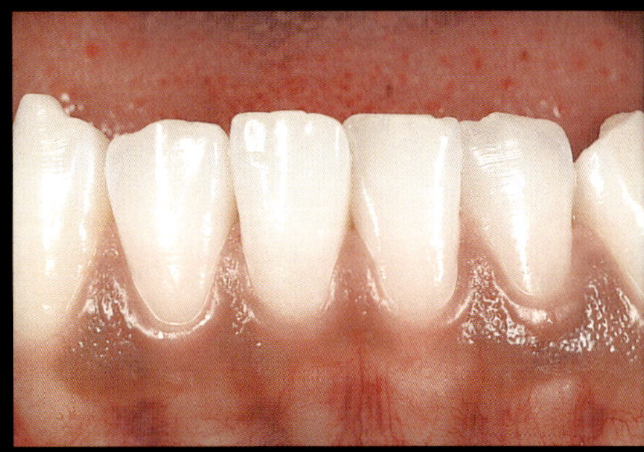

28-year-old female

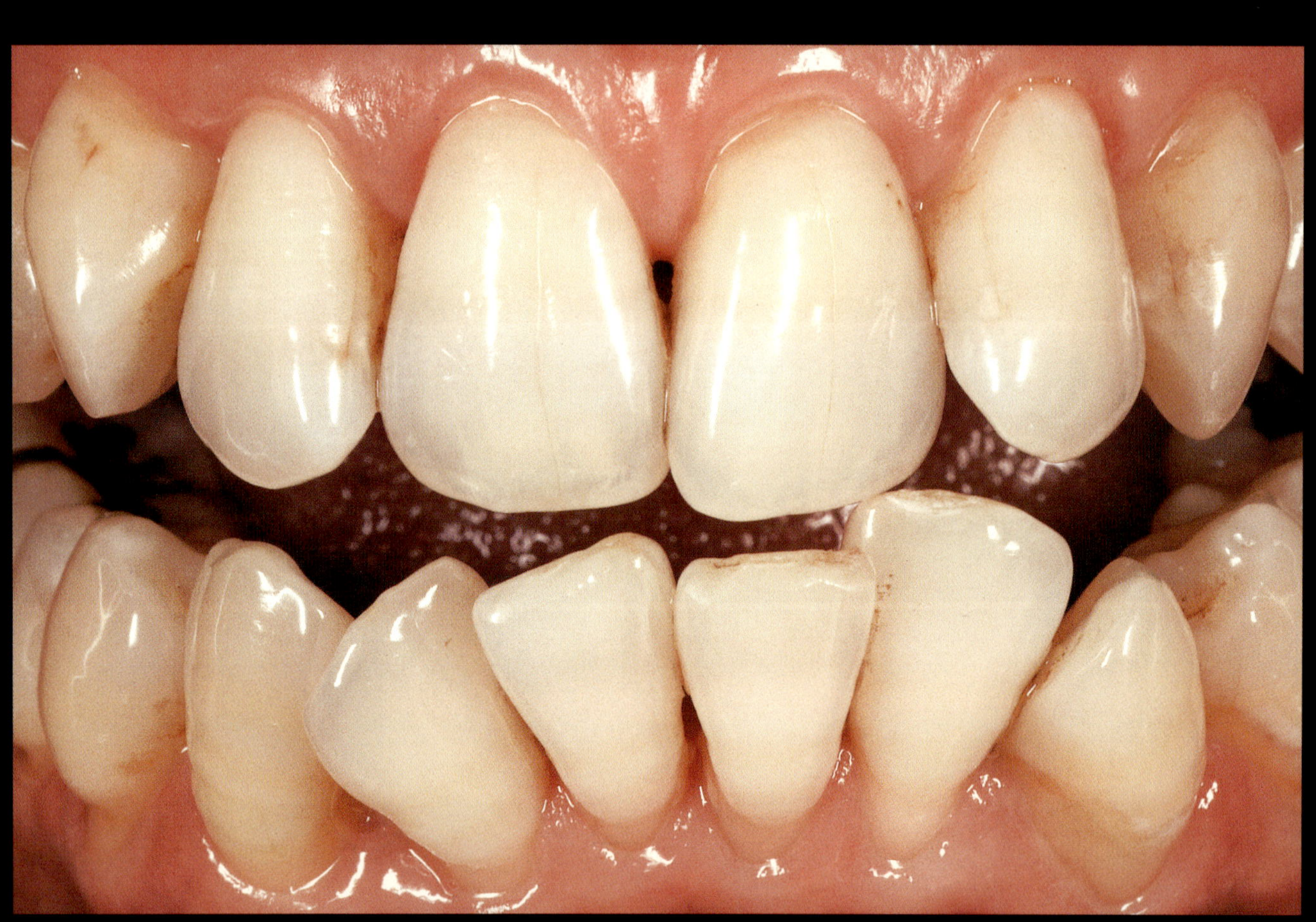

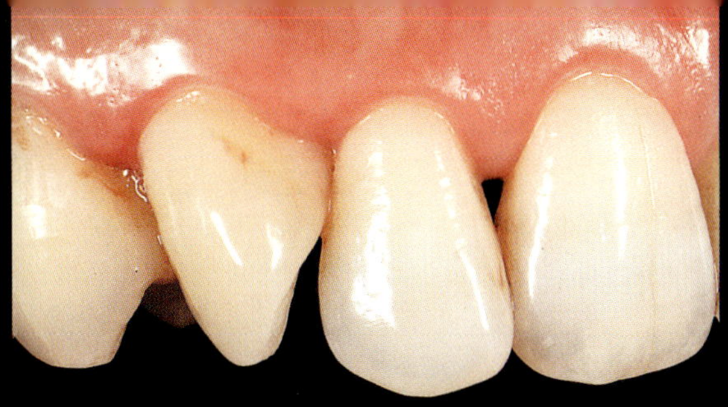
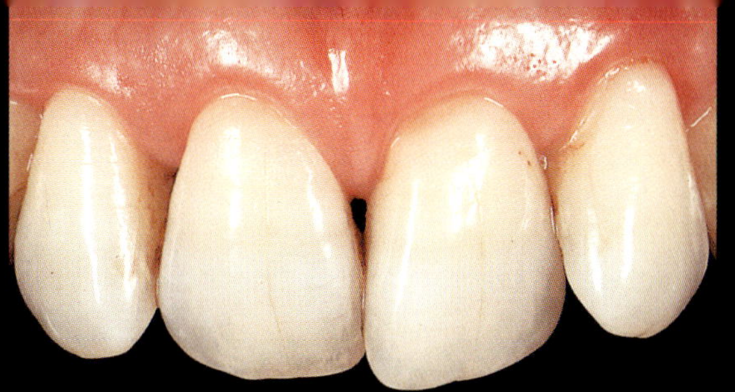
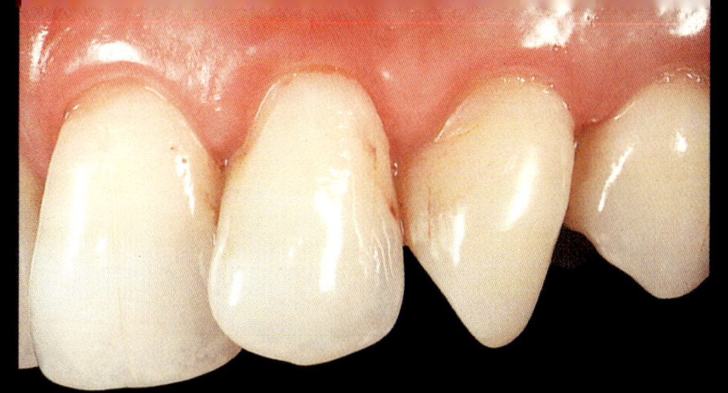
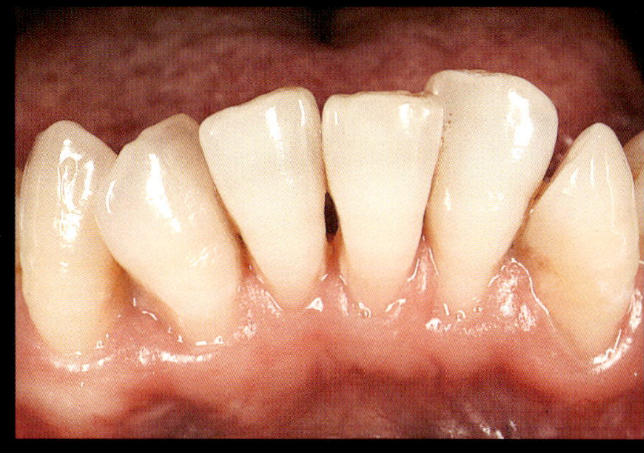

50-year-old female

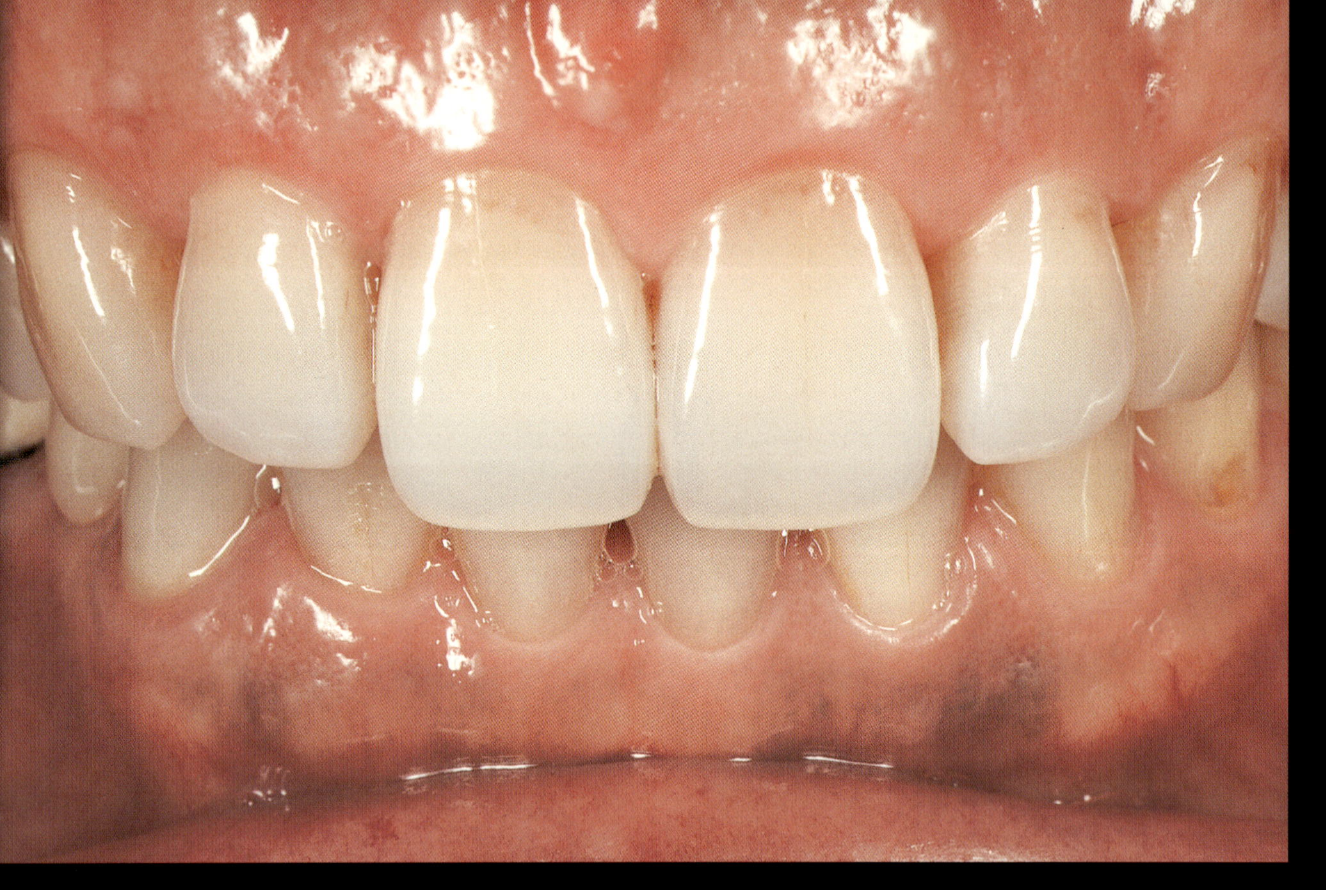

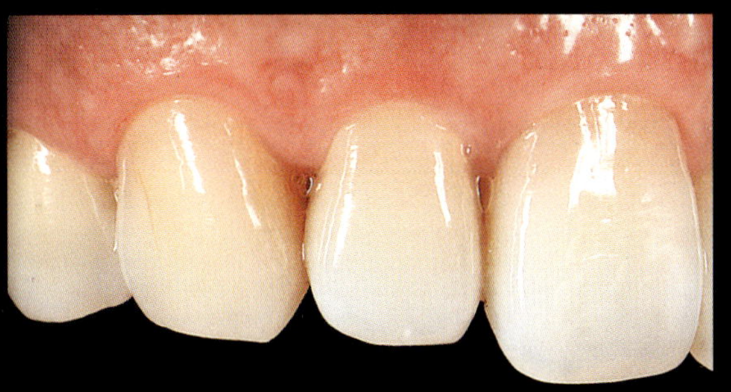
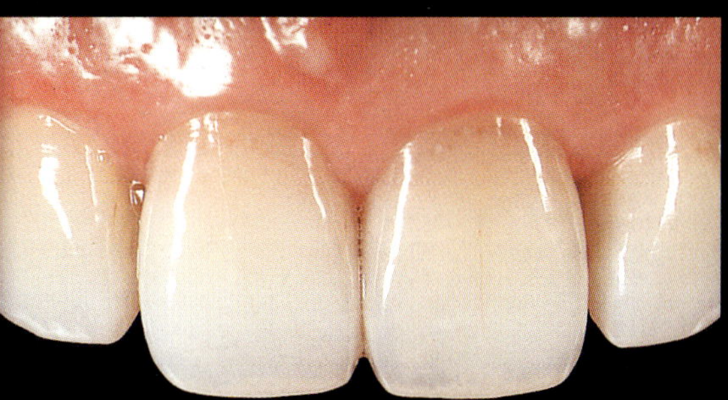
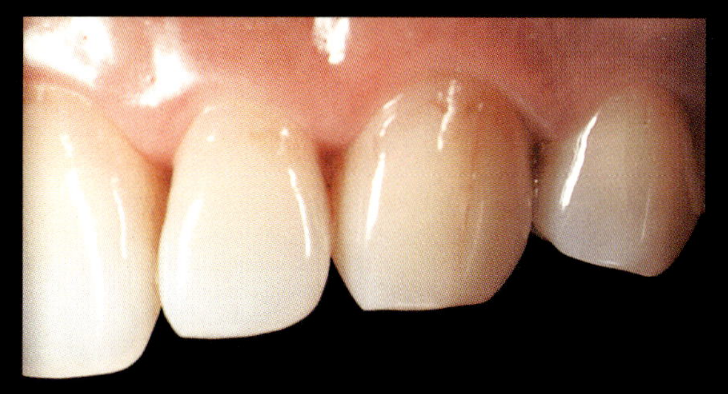
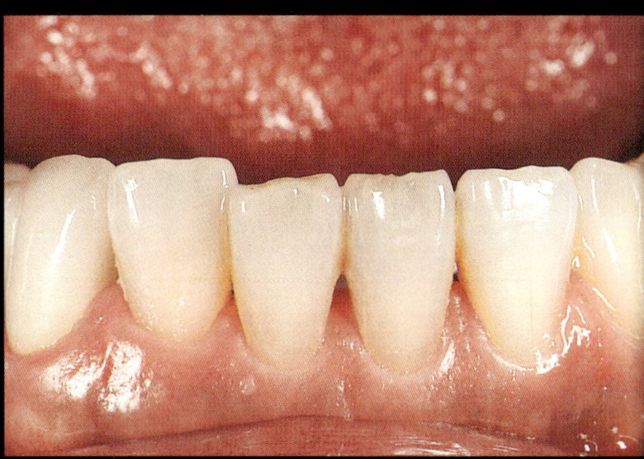

55-year-old female

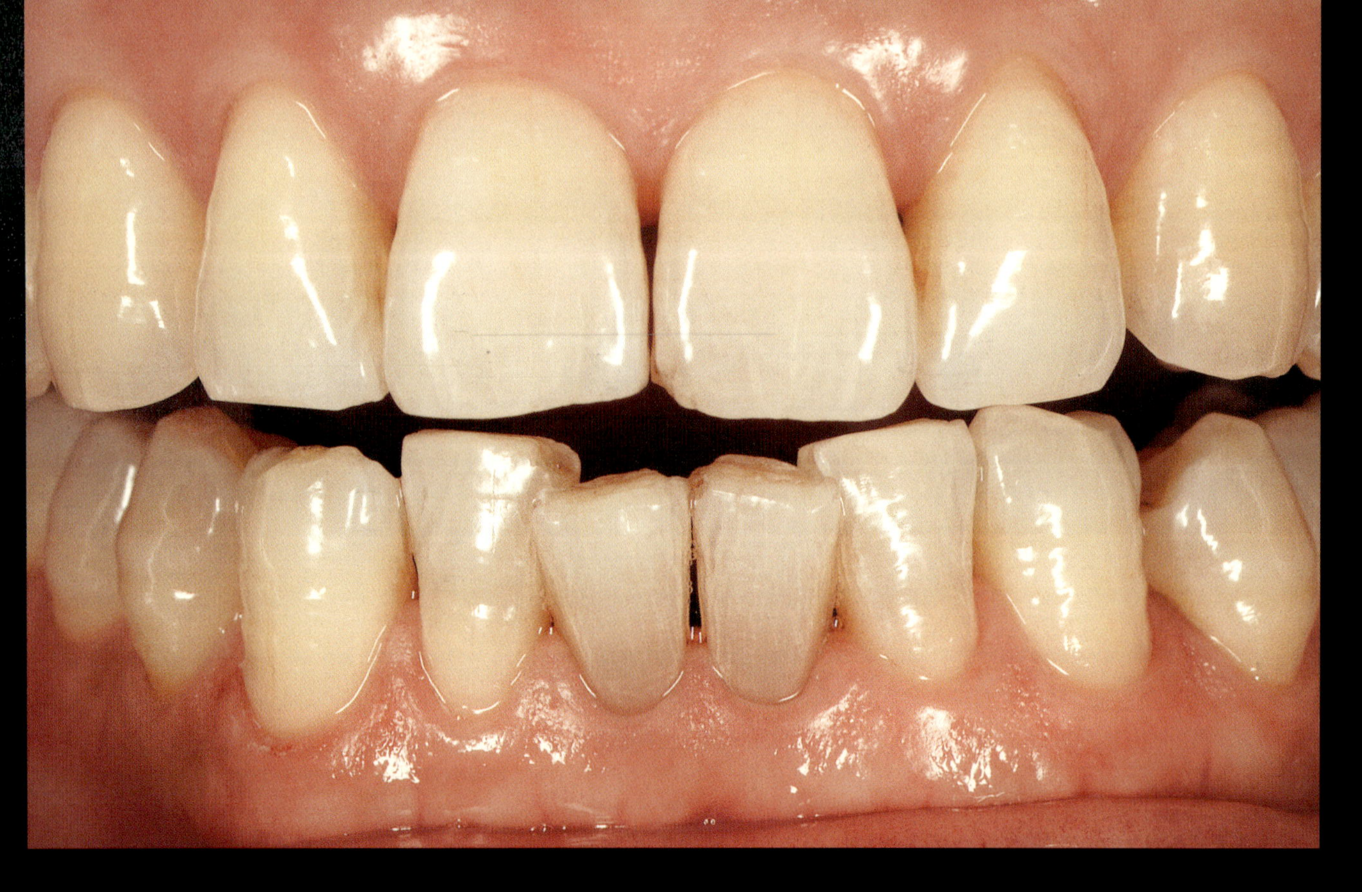

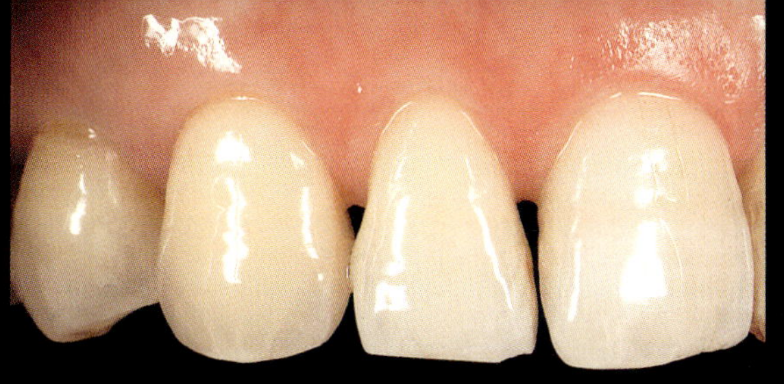
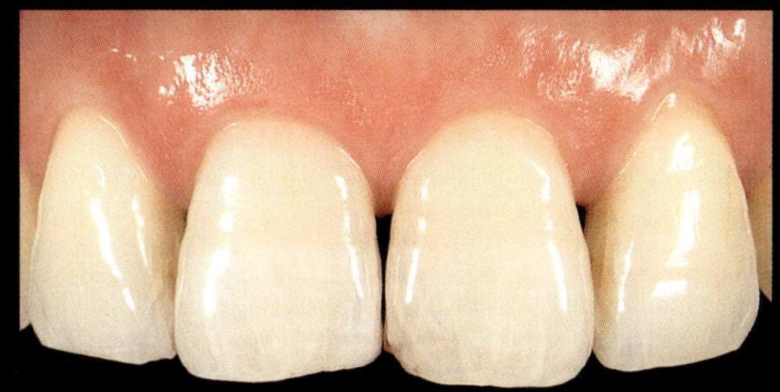
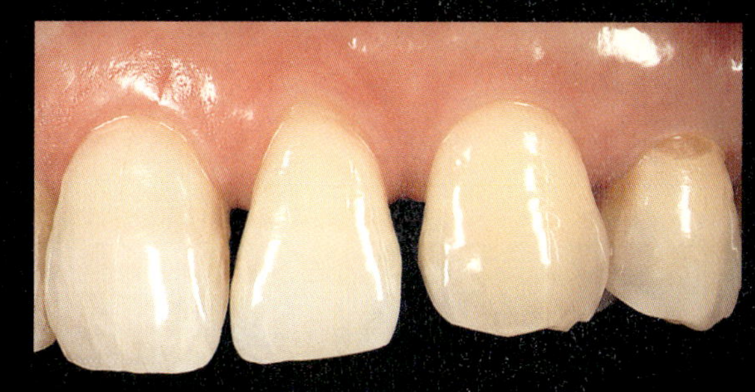
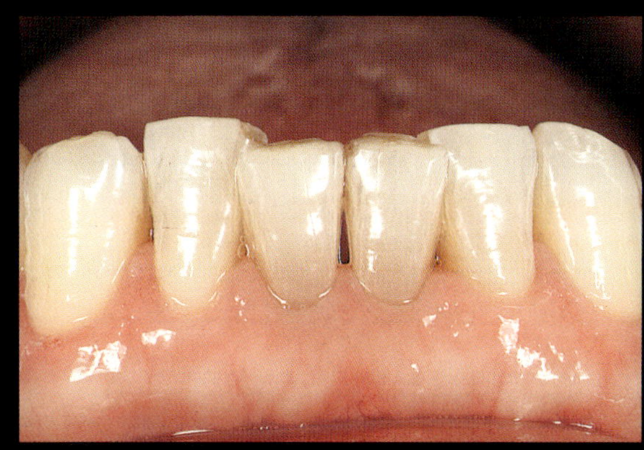

70-year-old female

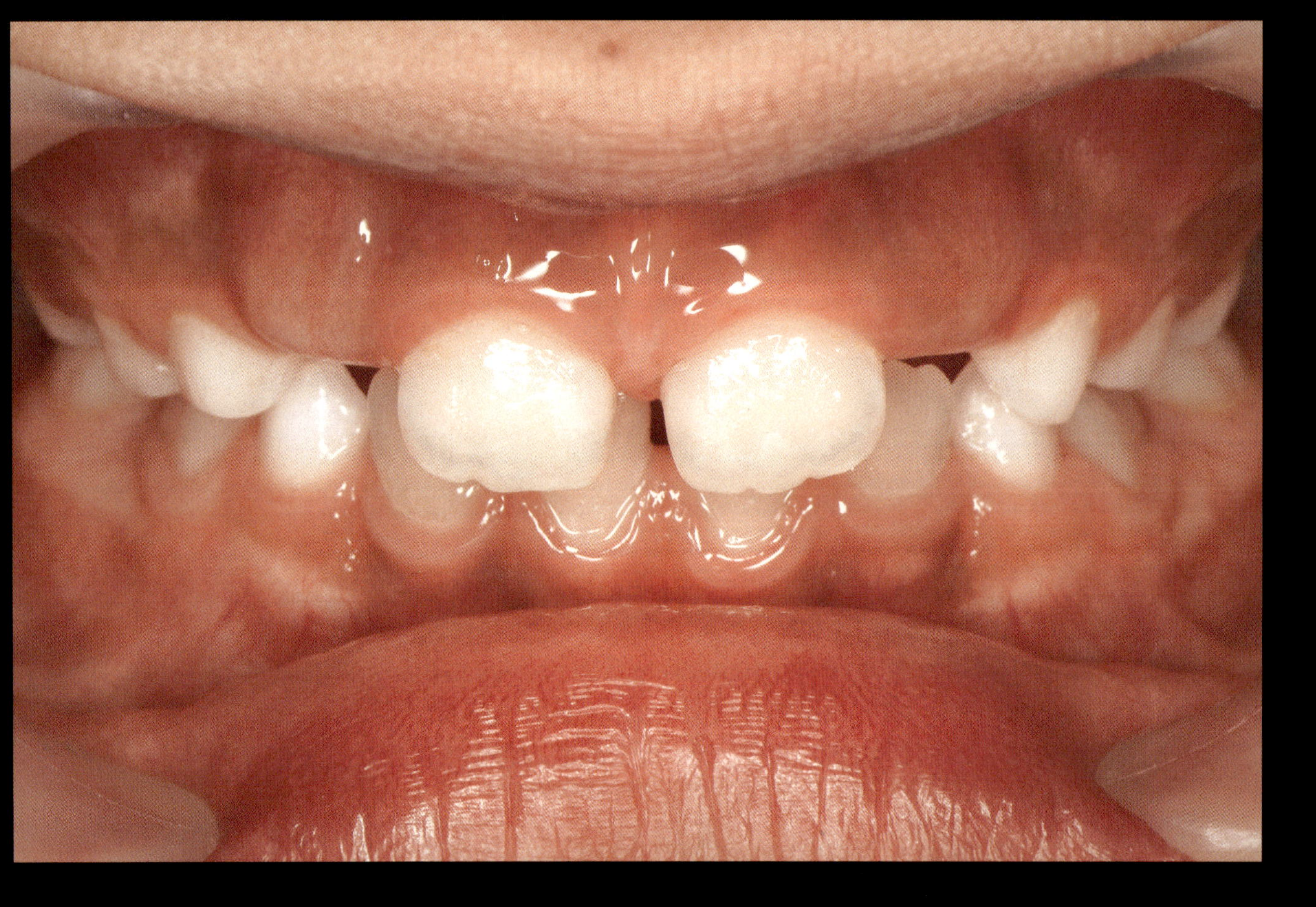

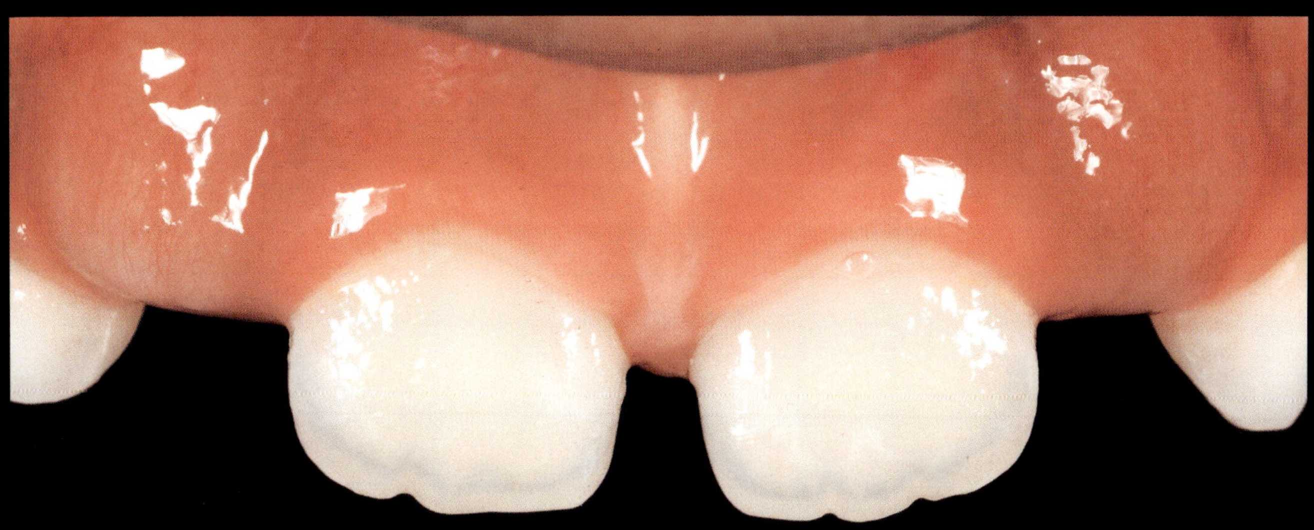

7-year-old male

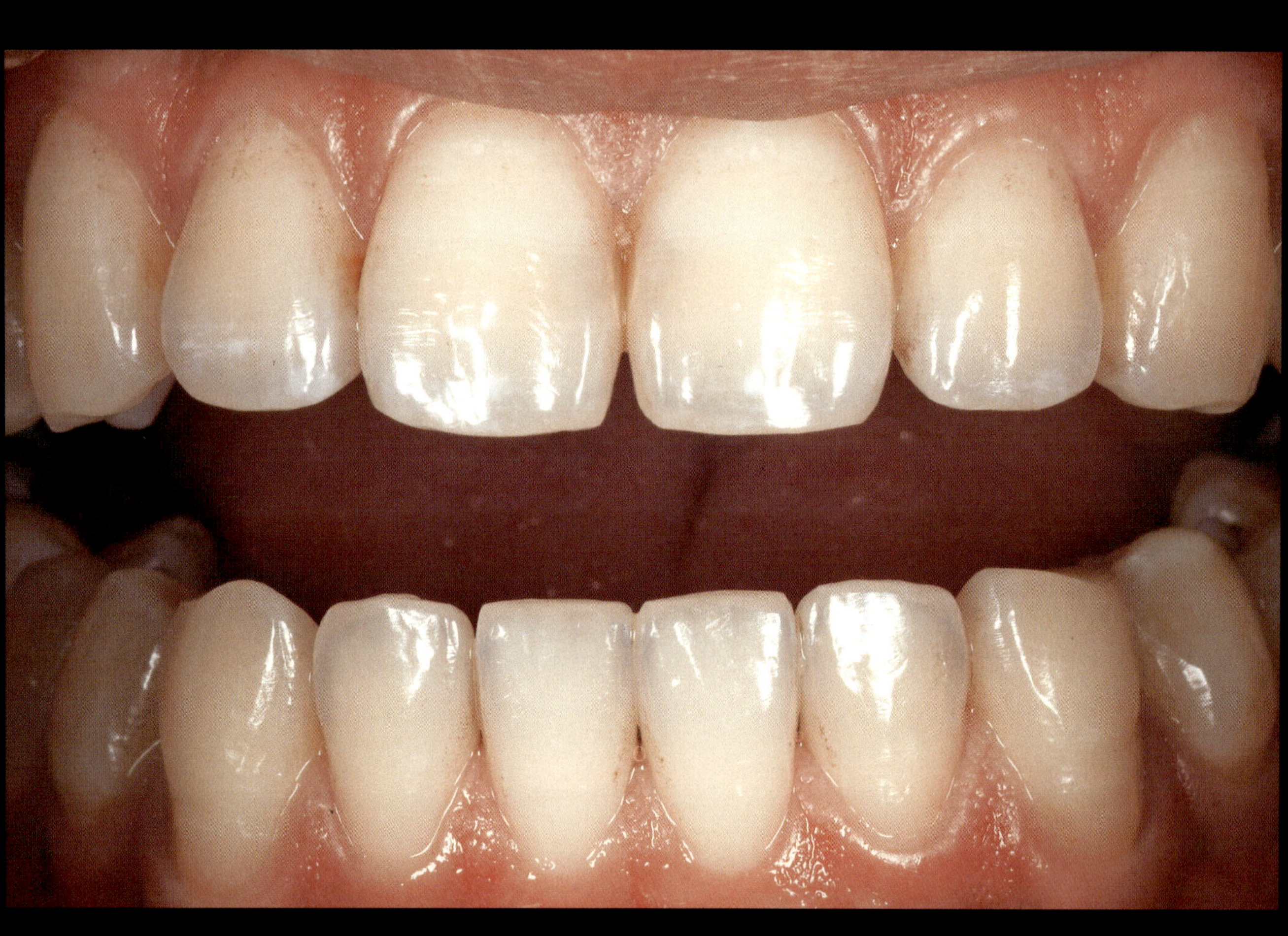

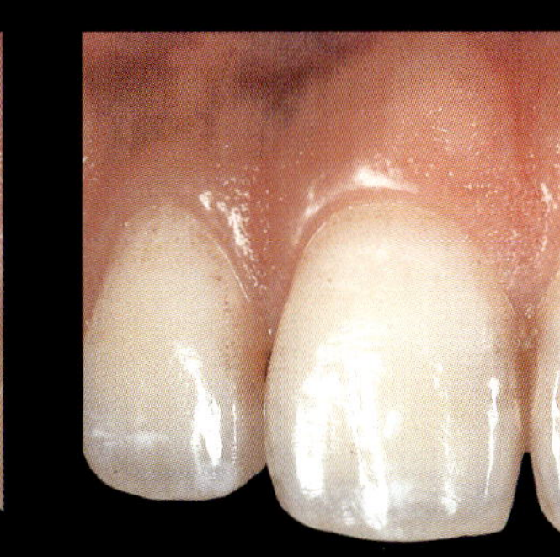

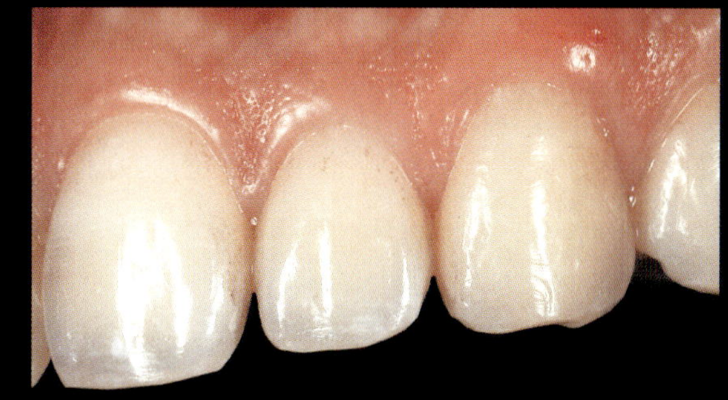

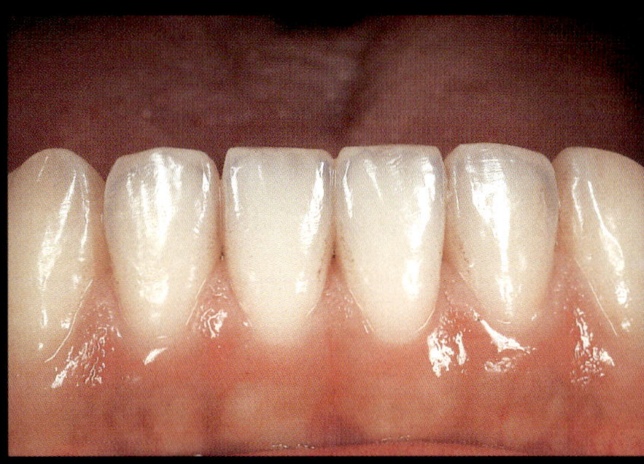

18-year-old male

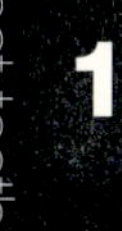

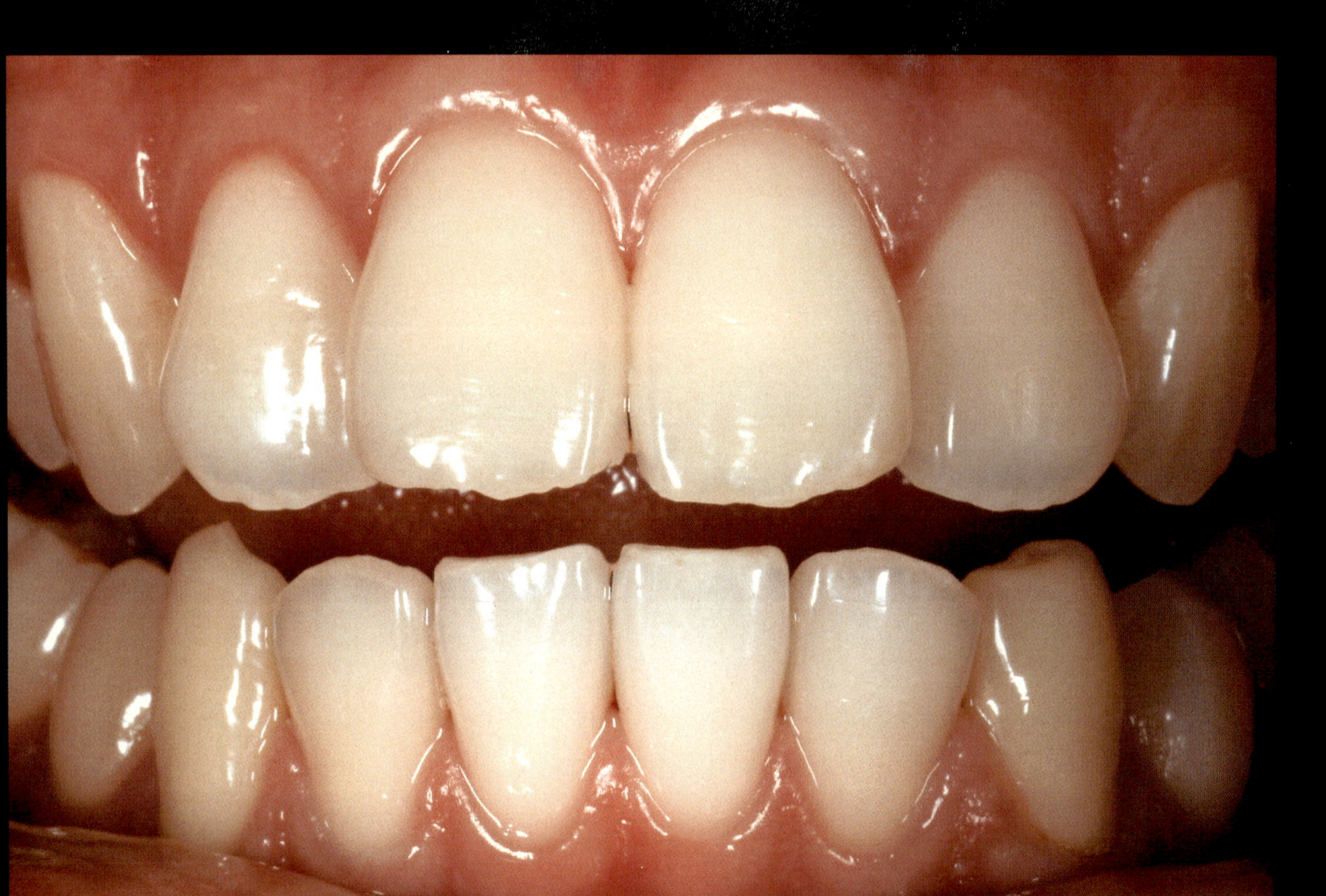

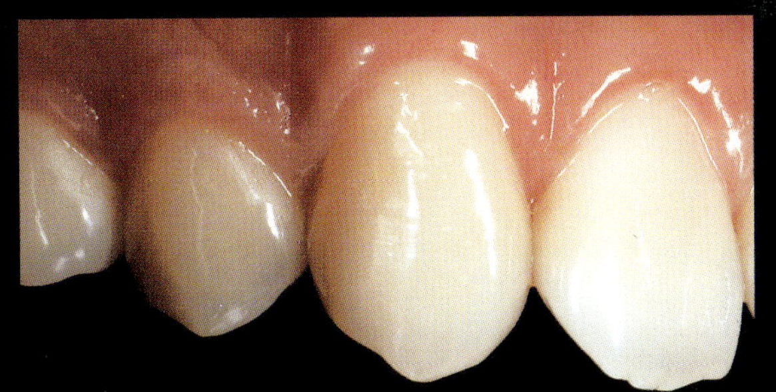

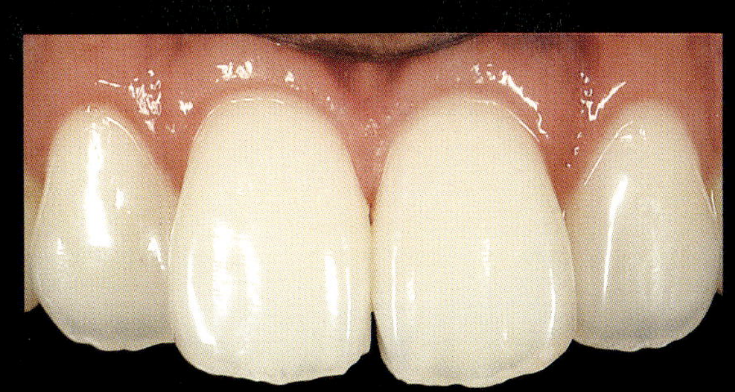

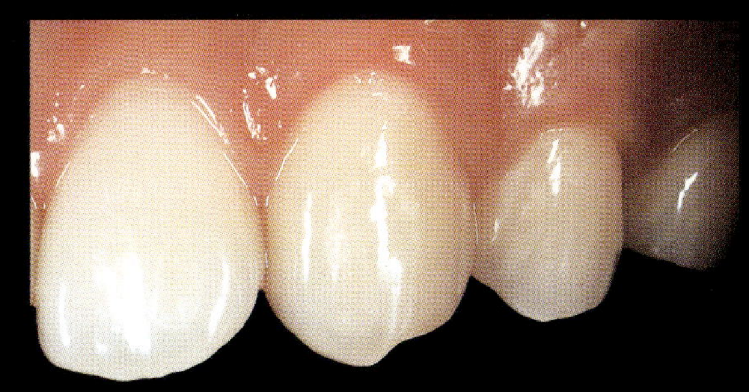

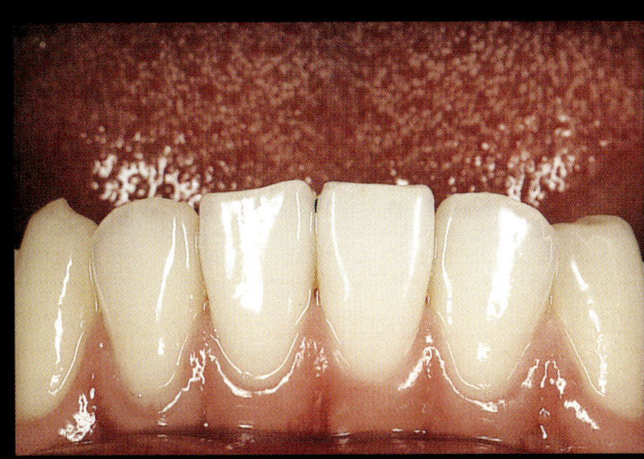

26-year-old male

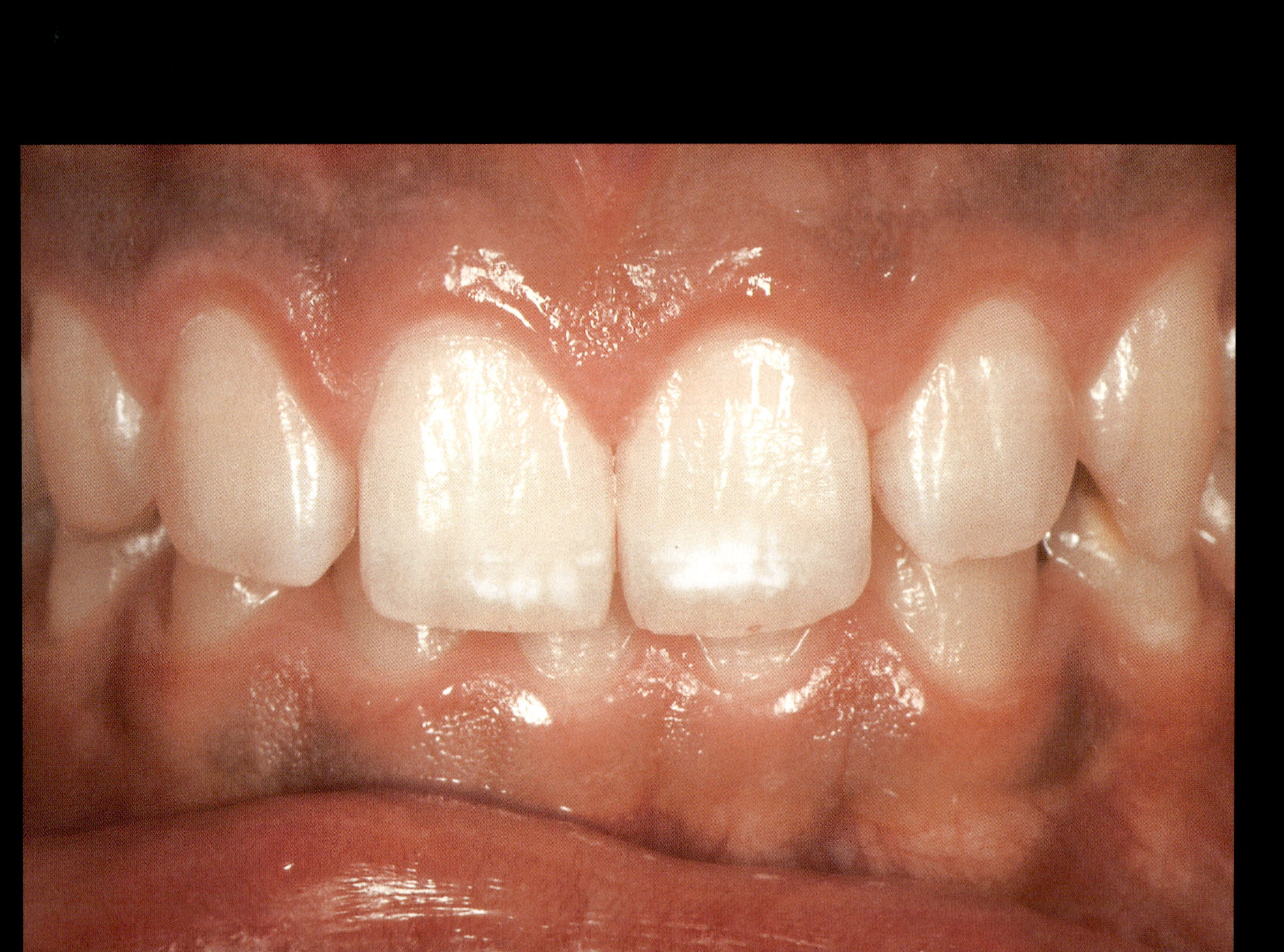

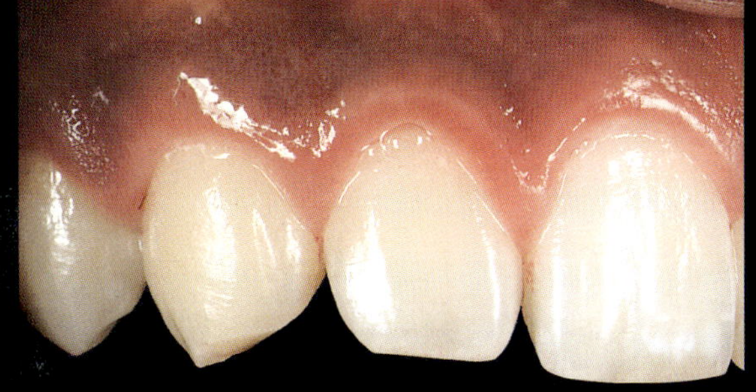

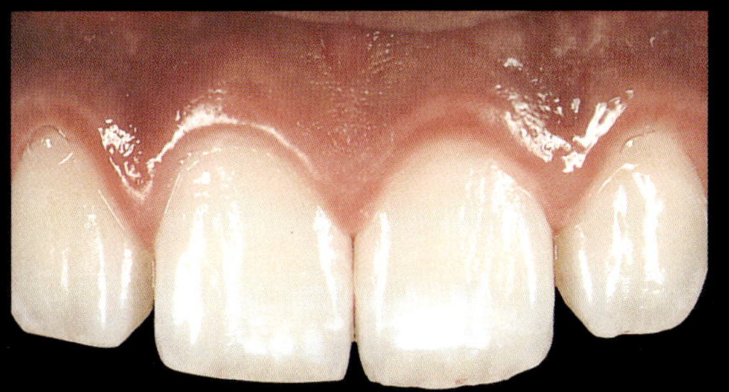

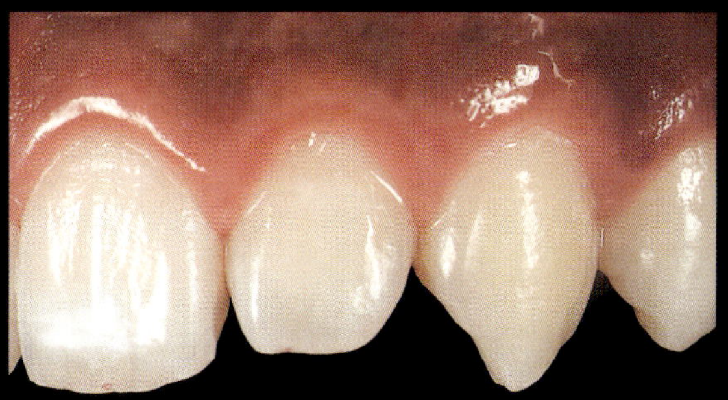

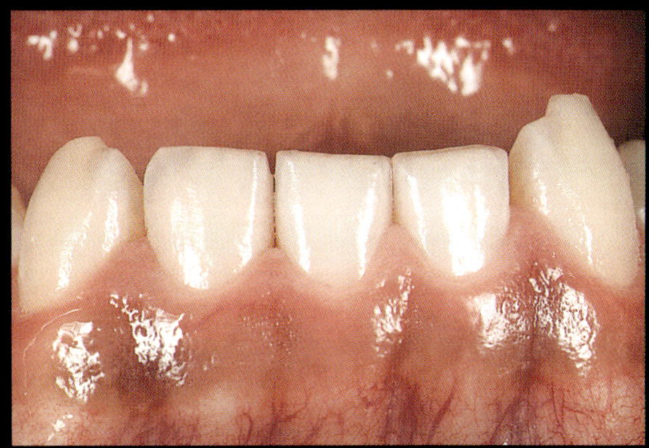

29-year-old male

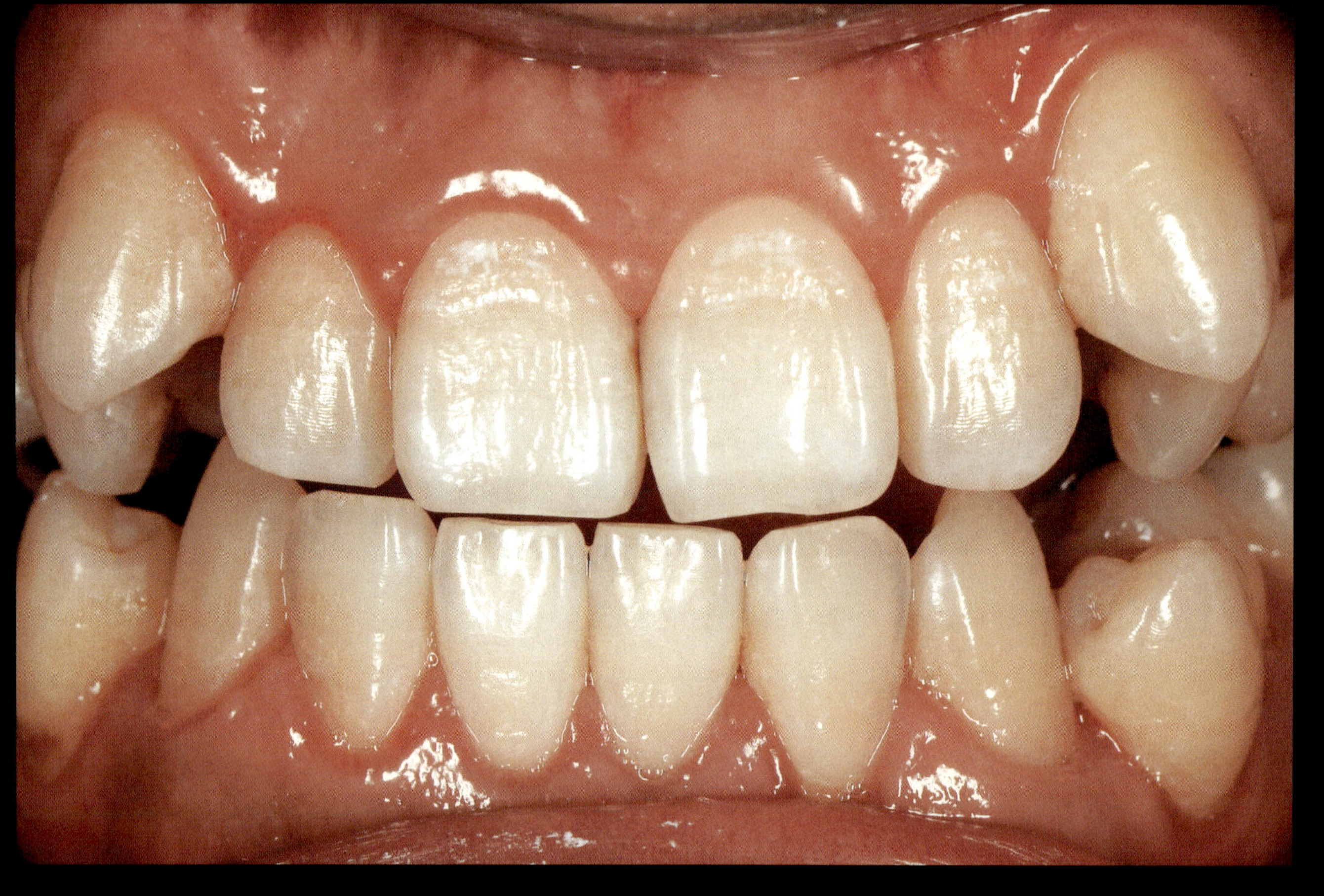

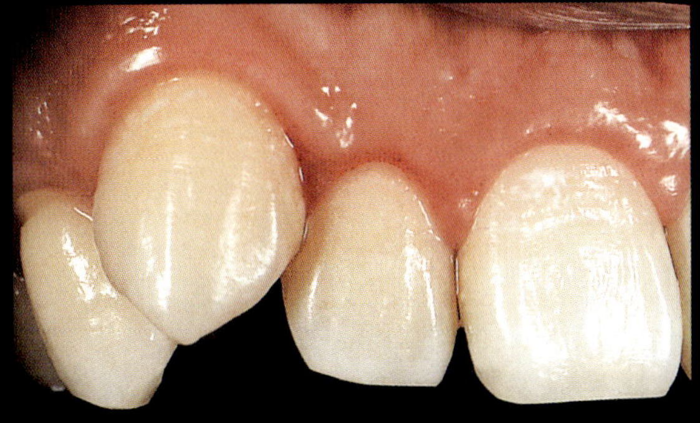
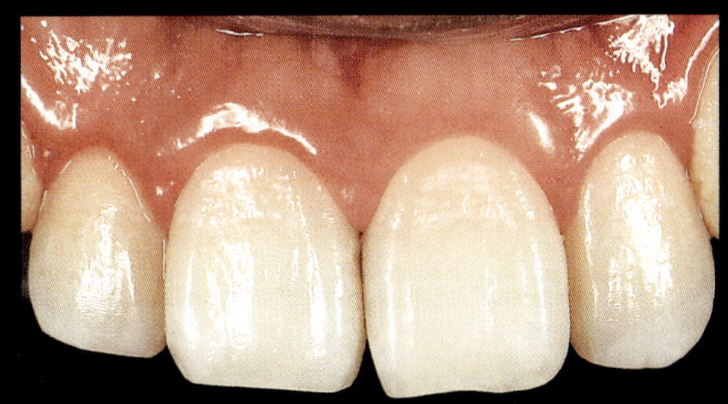
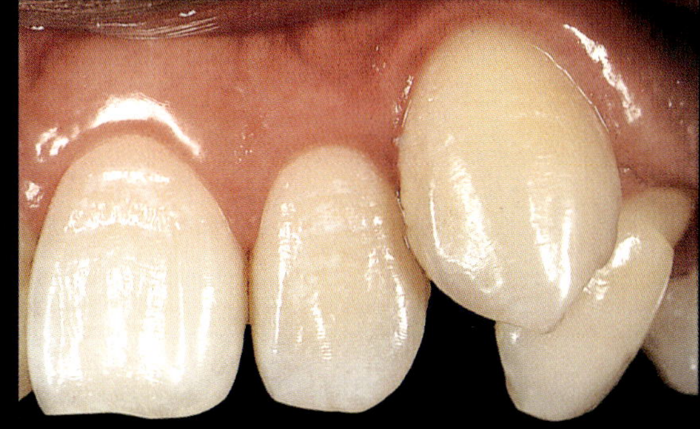
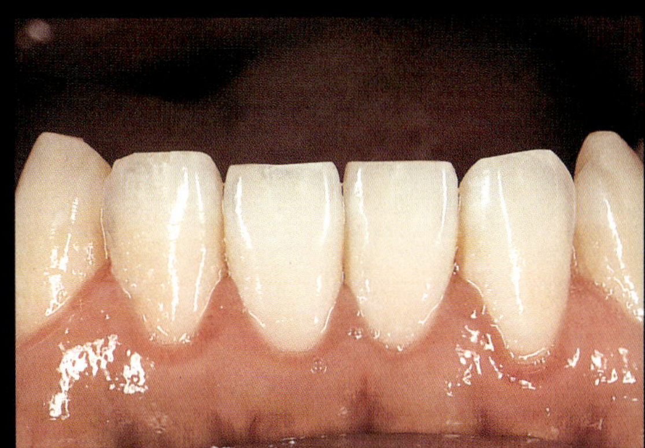

29-year-old male

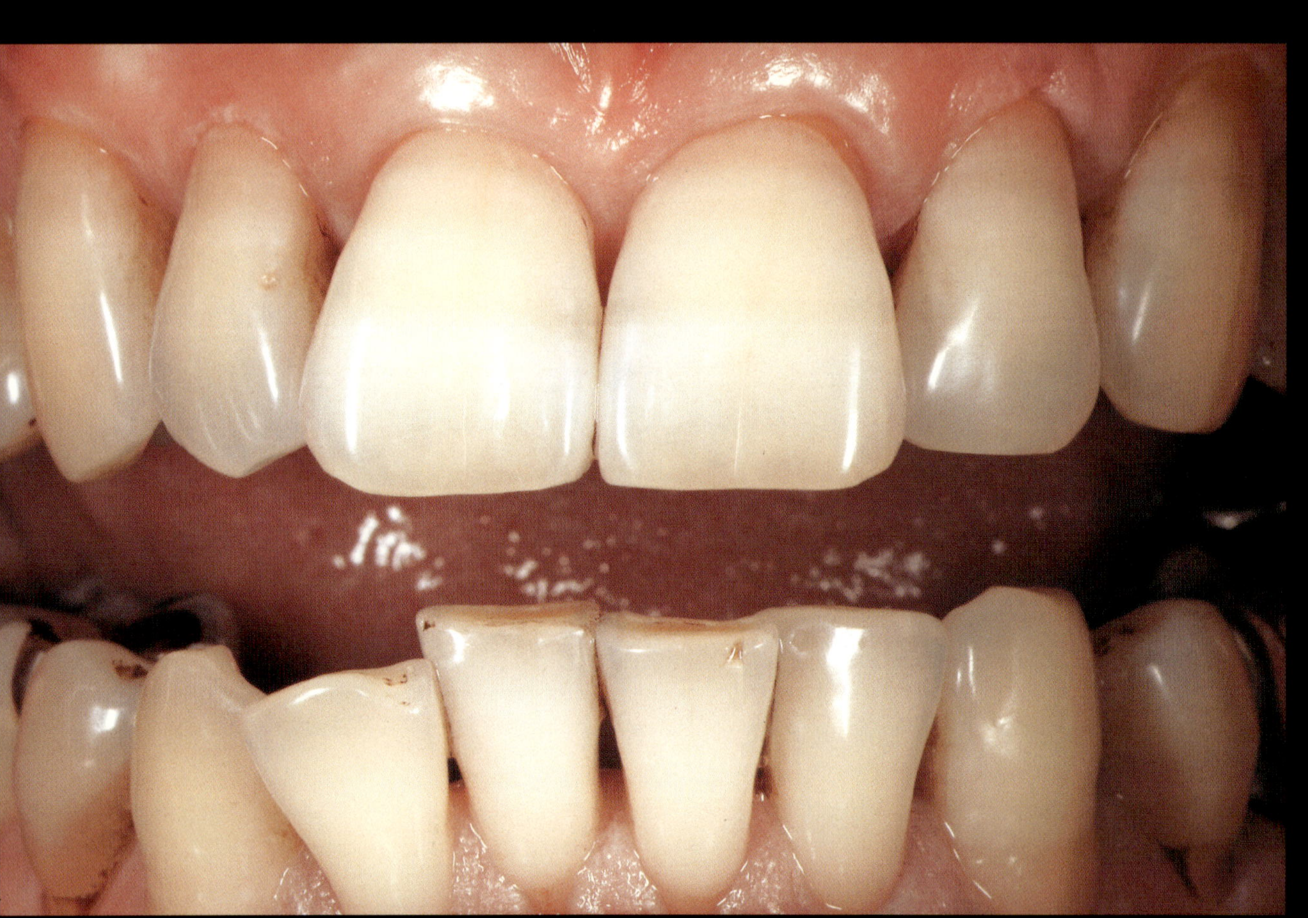

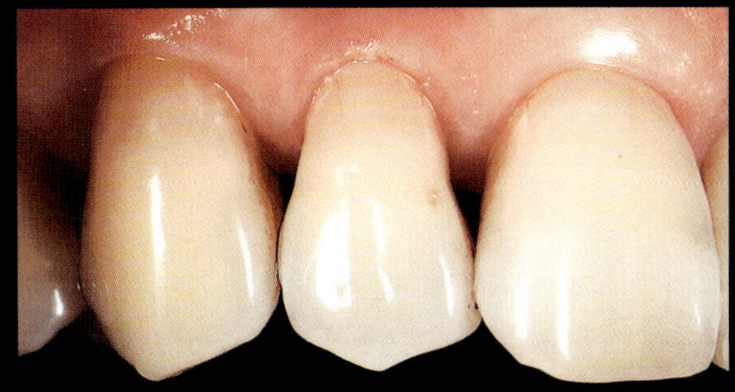
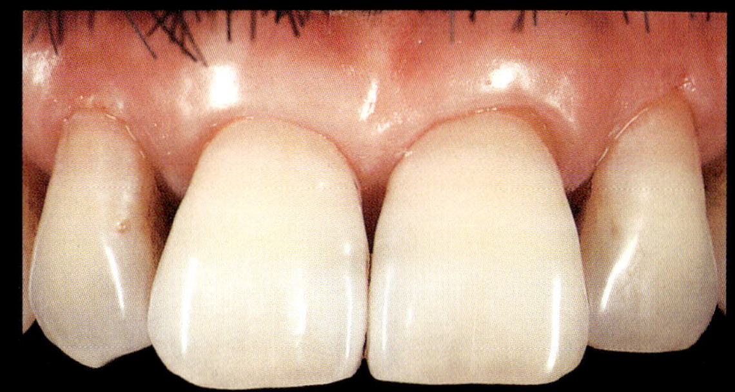
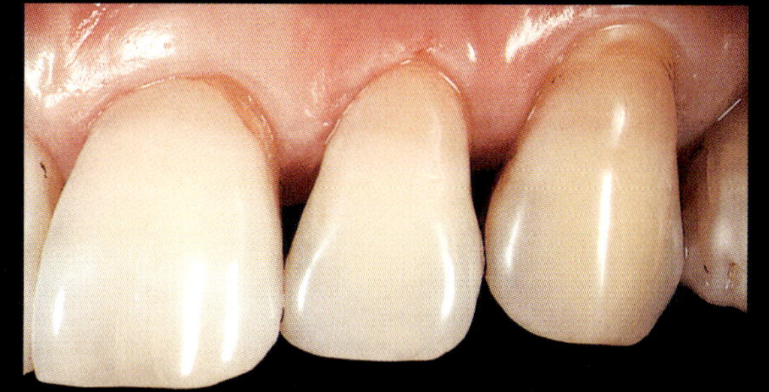
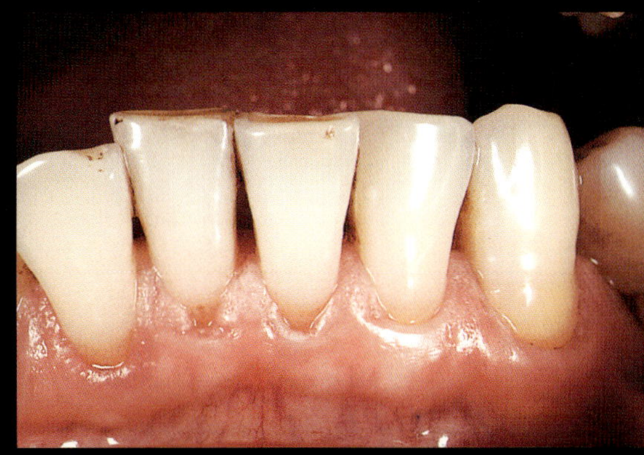

40-year-old male

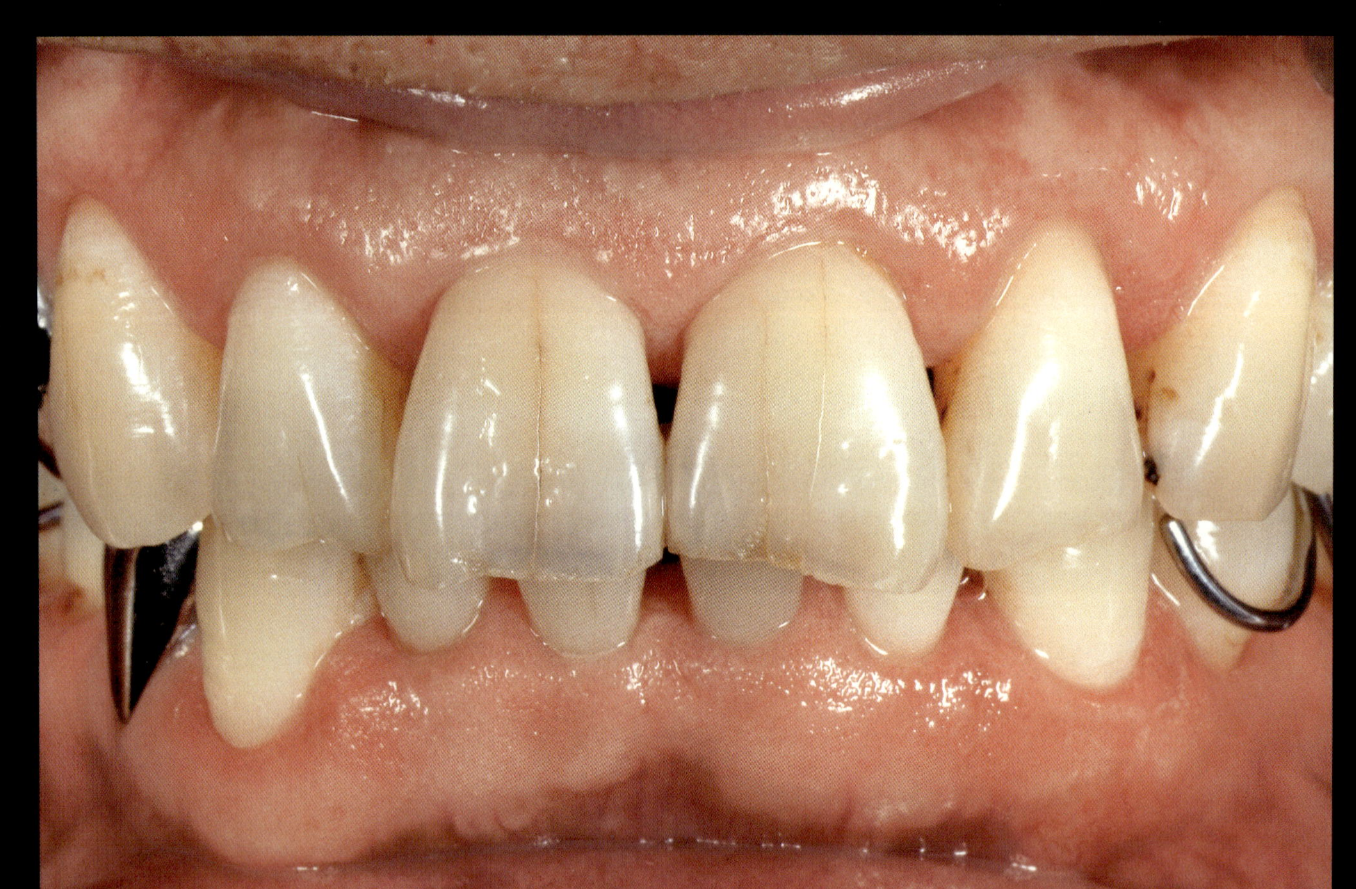

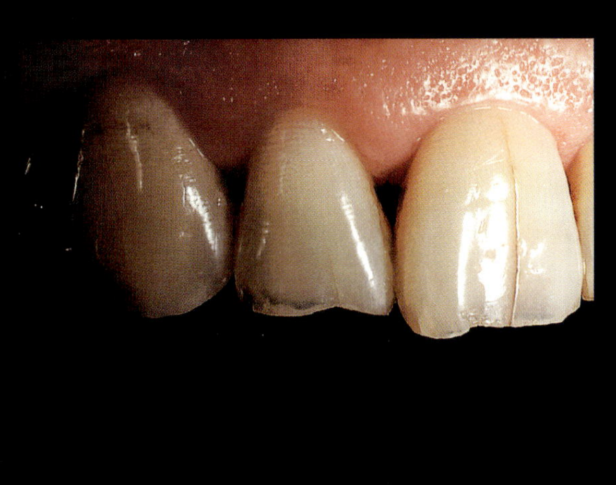
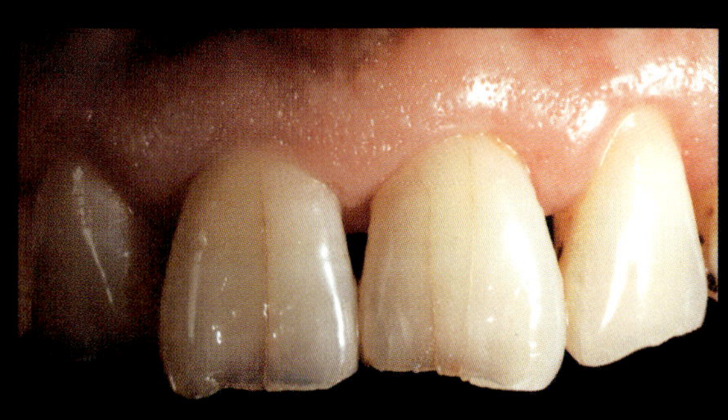
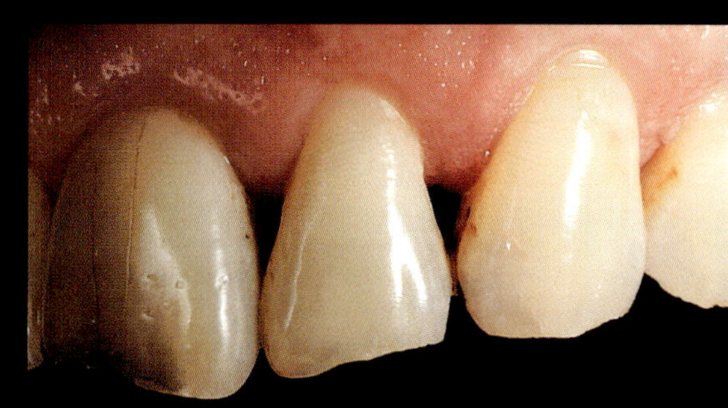
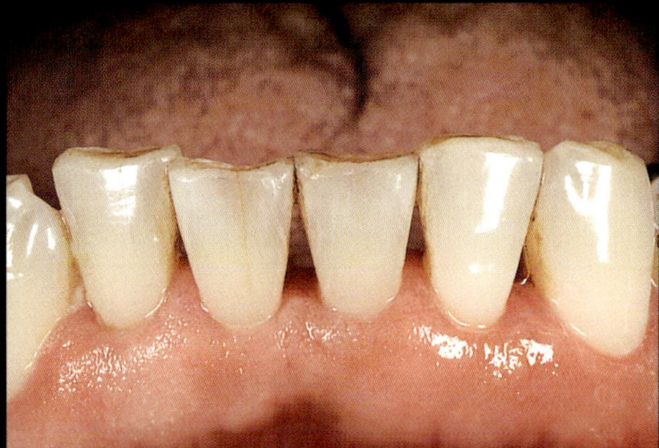

62-year-old male

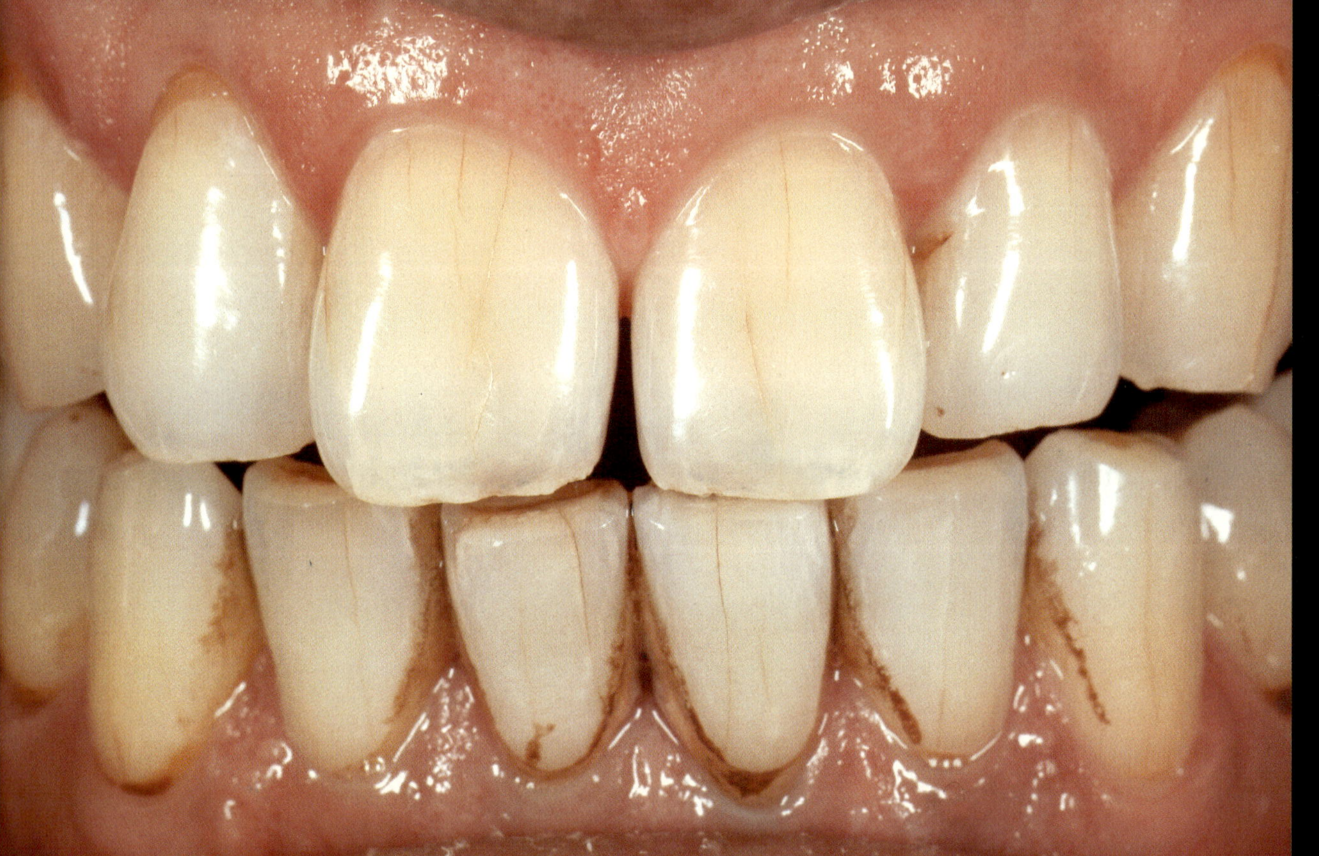

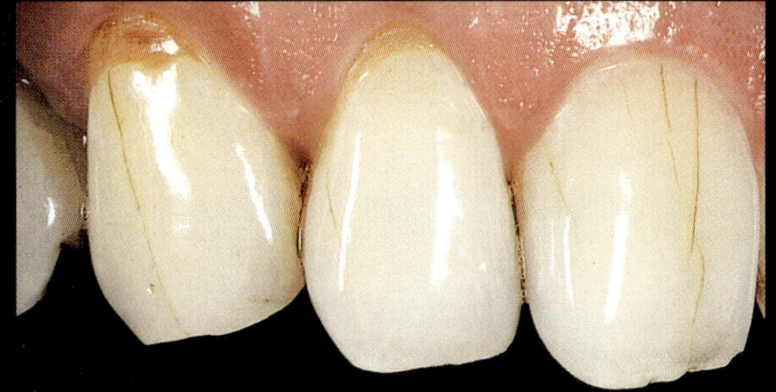
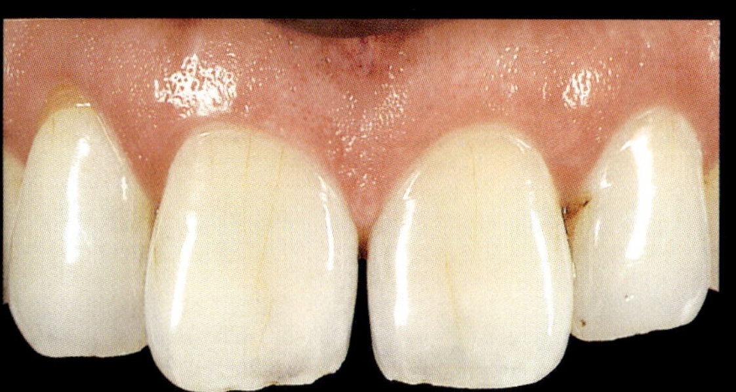
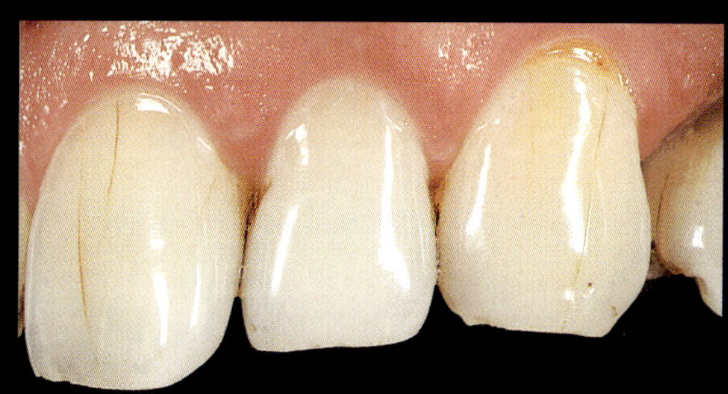
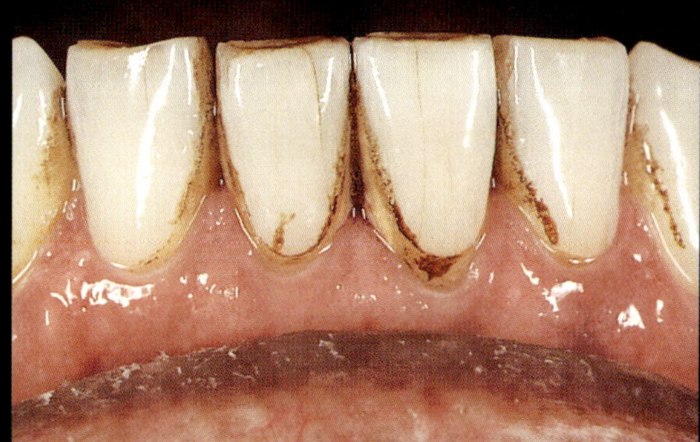

67-year-old male

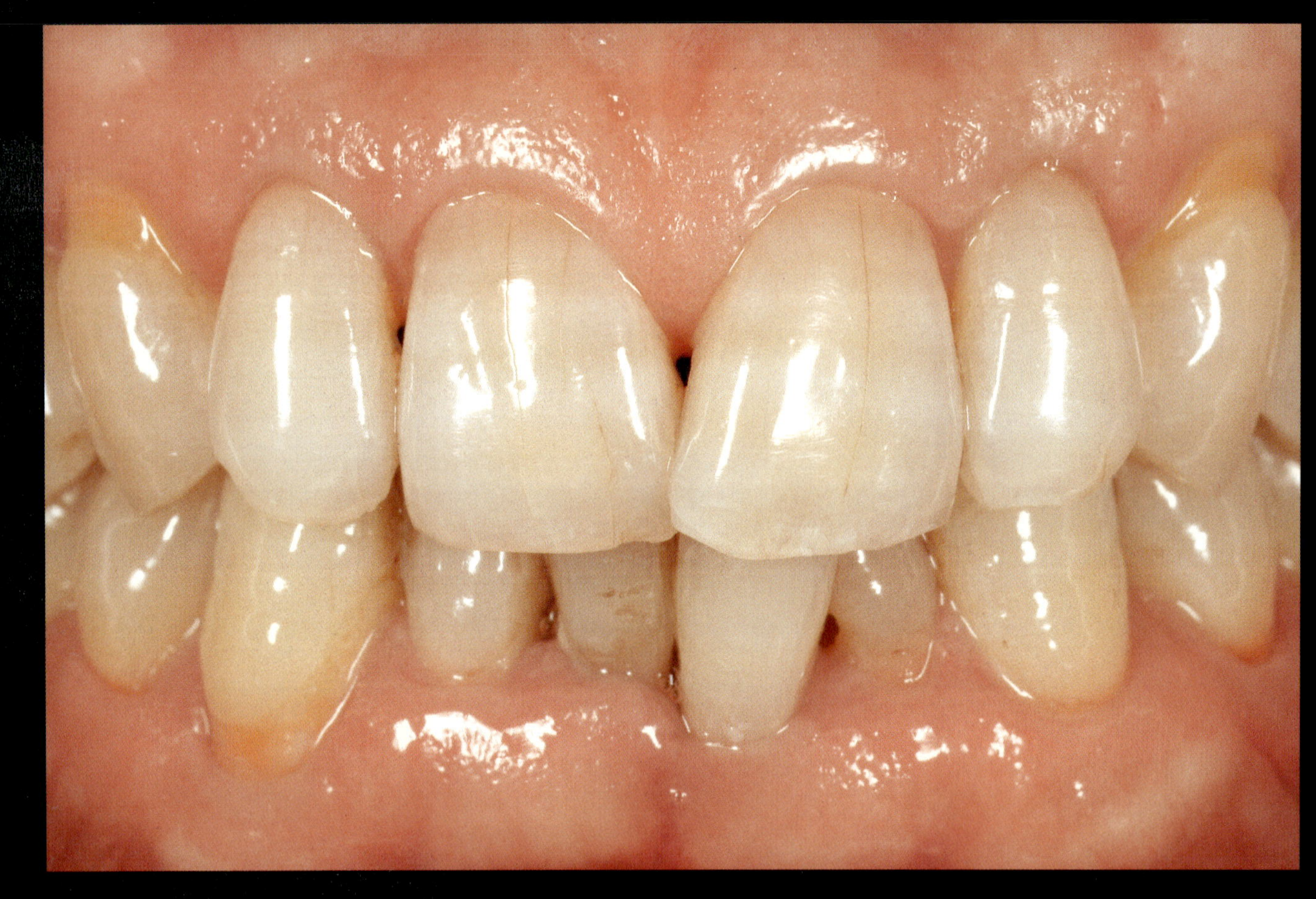

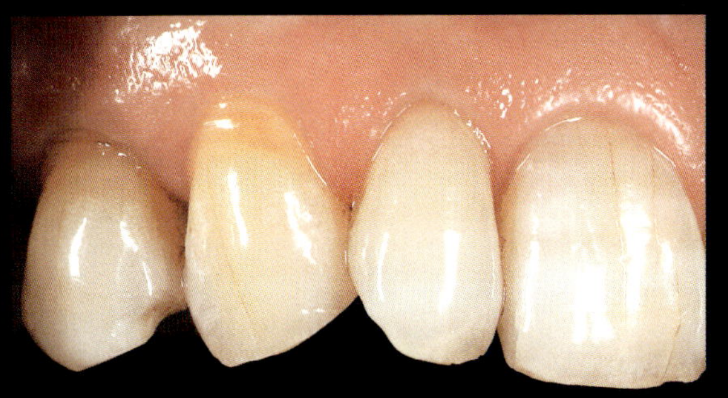
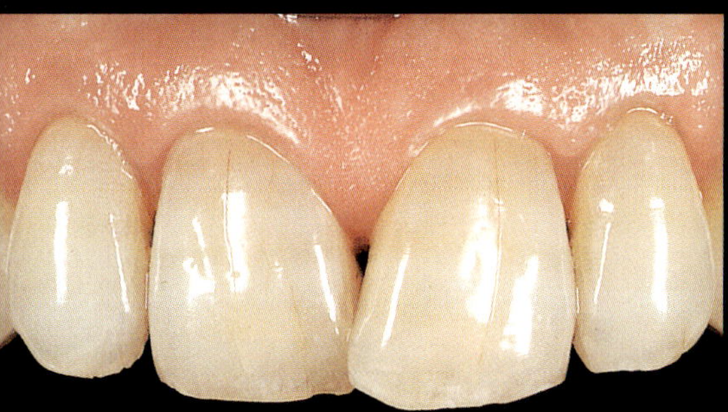
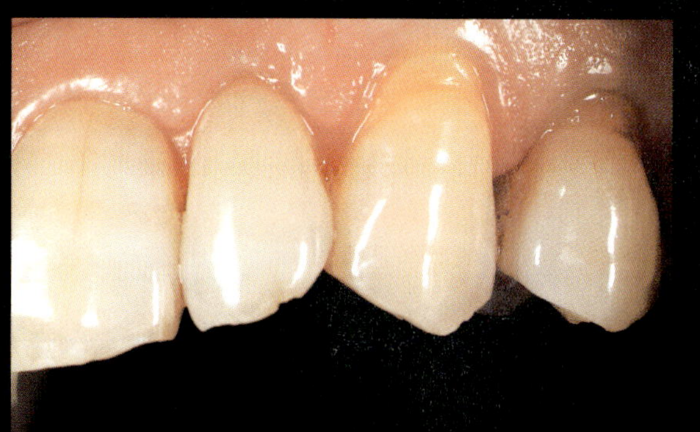
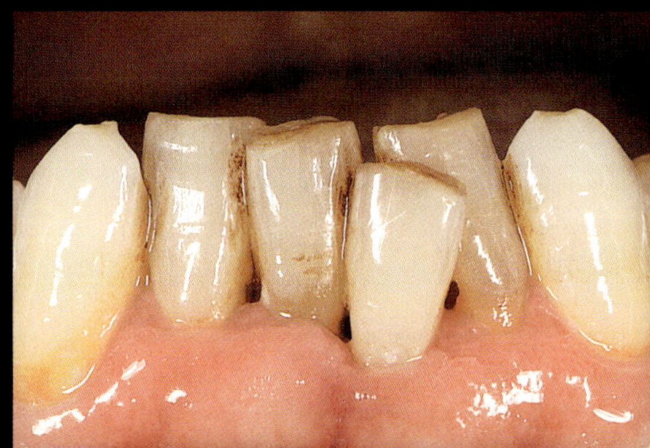

70-year-old male

References

1. Hidaka T, Masahiro M. Behandlungsgrundsätze zur Wiederherstellung der Zahnkrone. Tokio: Ishiyaku, 2003
2. Ricketts RM. Planning treatment on the basis of the facial pattern and an estimate of its growth. Angle Orthod 1952;27(1):14–37.
3. Diamond O. Facial Esthetics and Orthodontics. J Esthetic Dent 1996;8(3): 136–143.
4. Rufenacht C. Fundamentals of Esthetics. Chicago: Quintessence, 1990.
5. Fradeani M. Esthetic Rehabilitation in Fixed Prosthodontics. Chicago: Quintessence, 2004.
6. Hidaka T, Wakimoto Y. Zahnstellung. Teil 4: Ästhetik. Tokio: Quintessence, 2002:14–19.
7. Gargiulo A, Wentz F, Orban B. Dimensions and relations of the dentogingival junction in humans. J Periodontol 1961;32:261–267.
8. Nevins M, Skurow H. The intracrevicular restorative margin, the biologic width and the maintenance of the gingival margin. Int J Periodontics Restorative Dent 1984;4(3):30–49.
9. Lindhe J, Nyman S. Alteration of the position of the marginal soft tissue following periodontal surgery. J Clin Periodontol 1980;7(6):525–530.
10. Ericsson I, Lindhe J. Recession in sites with inadequate width of the keratinized gingiva. An experimental study in dog. J Clin Periodontol 1984;11(2):95–103.
11. Nevins M. Attached gingiva-mucogingival therapy and restorative dentistry. Int J Periodontics Restorative Dent 1986;6(4):9–27.
12. Maynard JG. Physiologic dimensions of the periodontium significant to the restorative dentist. J Periodontol 1979;50(4):170–174.
13. Maynard JG, Wilson RD. Diagnosis and management of mucogingival problems in children. Dent Clin North Am 1980;24(4):683-703.
14. Kois JC. Altering Gingival Levels: The Restorative Connection Part I: Biologic Variables. J Esthet Dent 1994;6(1):3–9.
15. Wennström JL. Mucogingival considerations in orthodontic treatment. Semin Orthod 1996;2(1):46-54.
16. Dragoo MR, Williams GB. Periodontal tissue reactions to restorative procedures. Part II. Int J Periodontics Restorative Dent 1982;2:35–45.
17. Carlsson L, Röstlund T, Albrektsson B, Albrektsson T, Brånemark P-I. Osseointegration of Titanium implants. Acta Orthop Scand 1986;57:285–289.
18. Weber HP, Buser D, Fiorellini JP, Williams RC. Radiographic evaluation of crestal bone levels adjacent to nonsubmerged titanium implants. Clin Oral Implants Res 1992;3(4):181–188.
19. Berglundh T, Lindhe J, Ericsson I, Marinello CP, Liljenberg B, Thomsen P. The soft tissue barrier at implants and teeth. Clin Oral Implants Res 1991;2(2):81–90.
20. Palacci P, Amenagement des tissus peri-implantaires intéret de la regeneration des papilles. Real Clin 1992;3:381–387.
21. Abrahamsson I, Berglundh T, Wennström J, Lindhe J. The peri-implant hard and soft tissues at different implant systems. A comparative study in the dog. Clin Oral Implants Res 1996;7(3):212–219.
22. Cochran DL, Hermann JS, Schenk RK, Higginbottom FL, Buser D. Biologic width around titanium implants. A histometric analysis of the implanto-gingival junction around unloaded and loaded nonsubmerged implants in the canine mandible. J Periodontol 1997;68(2):186–198.
23. Hermann JS, Cochran DL, Nummikoski PV, Beser D. Crestal bone changes around titanium implants. A radiographic evaluation of enloaded nonsubmerged and submerged implants in the canine mandible. J Periodontol 1997;68(11):1117–1130.
24. Salama H, Salama MA, Garber D, Adar P. The interproximal height of bone: a guidepost to predictable aesthetic strategies and soft tissue contours in anterior tooth replacement. Pract Periodontics Aesthet Dent 1998;10(9):1131–1141.
25. Phillips K, Kois JC. Aesthetic peri-implant site development: The restorative connection. Dent Clin North Am 1998;42(1):57–70.
26. Saadoum AP, Legall M, Touai B. Selection and ideal tridimensional implant position for soft tissue aesthetics. Pract Periodontics Aesthet Dent 1999;11(9):1063–1072.
27. Tarnow DP, Cho SC, Wallace SS. The effect of inter-implant distance on the height of inter-implant bone crest. J Periodontol 2000;71(4):546–549.
28. Small PN, Tarnow D. Gingival recession around implants: a 1-year longitudinal prospective study. Int J Oral Maxillofac Implants 2000;15(4):527–532.
29. Grunder U. Stability of the mucosal topography around single-tooth implants and adjacent teeth: 1-year results. Int J Periodontics Restorative Dent 2000; 20(1):11–17.
30. Garber DA, Salama MA, Salama H. Immediate Total Tooth Replacement. Compend Contin Educ Dent 2001;22(3):210–216, 218.
31. Palacci P. Esthetic Implant Dentistry: Soft and Hard Tissue Management. Chicago: Quintessence, 2001.
32. Giannopoulou C, Bernard JP, Buser D, Carrel A, Belser UC. Effect of intracrevicular restoration margins on peri-implant health: clinical, biochemical, and microbiologic findings around esthetic implants up to 9 years. Int J Oral Maxillofac Implants 2003;18(2):173–181.
33. Priest G. Predictability of soft tissue from around single-tooth implant restorations. Int J Periodontics Restorative Dent 2003;23:19–27.

34. Kan JYK, Rungcharassaeng K, Lozada J. Immediate placement and provisionalization of maxillary anterior single implants: 1-year prospective study. Int J Oral Maxillofac Implants 2003;18:31–39.
35. Kan JYK, Rungcharassaeng K. Interimplant papilla preservation in the esthetic zone: a report of six consecutive cases. Int J Oral Maxillofac Implants 2003;23(3):249–259.
36. Kan JYK, Rungcharassaeng K, Umezu K, Kois JC. Dimensions of peri-implant mucosa: an evaluation of maxillary anterior single implants in humans. J Periodontol 2003;74(4):557–562.
37. Tarnow T, Elian N, Flecher P, Froum S, Magner A, Cho S-C, Salama M, Salama H, Garber D. Vertical distance from the crest of bone to the height of the interproximal papilla between adjacent implants. J Periodontol 2003;74(12):1785–1788.
38. Covani U, Barone A, Cornelini R, Crespi R. Soft tissue healing around implants placed immediately after tooth extraction: a clinical report. Int J Oral Maxillofac Implants 2004;19(4):549–553.
39. Bianchi AE, Sanfilippo F. Single-tooth replacement by immediate implant and connective tissue graft: a 1-9-year clinical evaluation. Clin Oral Implants Res 2004;15(3):269–277.
40. Pilkington EL. Esthetics and optical illusions in dentistry. J Am Dent Assoc 1936;23:641–651.
41. Albers HF. Tooth-Colored Restoratives, Principles and Techniques. Hamilton: BC Decker, 92002.
42. Magne P, Belser Urs. Bonded Porcelain Restorations. Chicago: Quintessence, 2002.
43. Ishihara M. Einfluss der Zahnsubstanz devitaler Zähne mit aufgebautem Pfeiler auf Fraktur und Verlaufsrichtung der Fraktur. Tsurumi-schigaku (Bericht der zahnmedizinischen Fachgesellschaft der Tsurumi University, Institut für Zahnmedizin) 1998;24(1):157–170.
44. Mannocci F, Ferrari M, Watson TF. Intermittent loading of teeth restored using quartz fiber, carbon-quartz fiber, and zirconium dioxide ceramic root canal posts. J Adhesive Dent 1999;1(2):153–158.
45. Schwickerath H. Werkstoffprüfung von Vollkeramiksystemen. In: Kappert HF (Hg) Vollkeramik: Wekstoffkunde - Zahntechnik - klinische Erfahrhung. Berlin: Quintessenz, 1996:87–102.
46. Wagner WC, Chu TM. Biaxial flexural strength and indentation fracture toughness of three dental core ceramics. J Prosthet Dent 1996;76(2):140–144.
47. Fischer H, Marx R. Lava Crowns and Bridges. 3M ESPE, 2004.

Bibliographic sources for illustrations marked with a red square ■

(Translation of original titles)

Page 6 Hidaka T. Treatment considerations for esthetic restorations – Guidelines for esthetic analysis and for the selection of restorative materials. Dental Diamond 2003; 28 (393):27
Page 28 Hidaka T. Aesthetic Dentistry, Hotetsu-rinsho, 2002;35(6):585
Page 41 Hidaka T. Treatment principles for crown restorations. Tokyo: Ishiyaku, 2003:109 (reprint from Hotetsu-rinsho)
Page 42 Hidaka T. Treatment principles for crown restorations. Tokyo: Ishiyaku, 2003:110–111 (reprint from Hotetsu-rinsho)
Page 43 Hidaka T. Treatment principles for crown restorations. Tokyo: Ishiyaku, 2003:109 (reprint from Hotetsu-rinsho)
Page 67 Hidaka T. Treatment considerations for esthetic restorations – Guidelines for esthetic analysis and for the selection of restorative materials. Dental Diamond 2003; 28(393):34
Page 69 Hidaka T. Treatment considerations for esthetic restorations – Guidelines for esthetic analysis and for the selection of restorative materials. Dental Diamond 2003;28(393):35
Page 69 Hidaka T. Treatment principles for crown restorations. Tokyo: Ishiyaku, 2003:52 (reprint from Hotetsu-rinsho)
Page 75 Hidaka T. Treatment principles for crown restorations. Tokyo: Ishiyaku, 2003:53 (reprint from Hotetsu-rinsho)
Page 81 Hidaka T. Prerequisites for the esthetic success of implant prostheses. Dental Diamond 2006;31(436):46
Page 93 Hidaka T. Preventive Periodontology. Tokyo: Ishiyaku, 2007:292
Page 95 Hidaka T. Preventive Periodontology. Tokyo: Ishiyaku, 2007:292